Neutrality Exercise Workbook AAMI

Acknowledgements	3
Introduction	4
Holistic Peer Counseling (HPC)	6
Getting Started with The Neutrality Exercise	7
A Basic Grounding	8
The Neutrality Exercise	11
Presencing	14
Introspection	15
The Entire Practice: Step by Step	16
Topic 1: Bubbles	22
Introspection	26
Topic 2: Skin to Skin	28
Introspection	33
Topic 3: Breastfeeding	35
Introspection	39
Topic 4: Hatted Newborn	41
Introspection	46
Topic 5: Gender Scan	48
Introspection	52
Topic 6: Preceptors	54
Introspection	59
Topic 7: Baby Baths	61
Introspection	65
Topic 8: Monitoring	67
Introspection	72
Topic 9: Formula	74
Introspection	78
Topic 10: Circumcision	80

Introspection	85
Topic 11: Schedule a Caesarean	87
Introspection	91
Topic 12: Local Obstetricians	93
Introspection	97
Topic 13: You Choose	99
Introspection	105
Topic 14: You Choose	107
Introspection	113
Topic 15: You Choose	115
Introspection	121
Bonus Practice	123
Thank you	125
A Note From The Author	126

Acknowledgments:

Thank you….

- To my family for loving me as me. I love you all so much!

- To Lori Barklage for being my midwife through out this project.

- To Christina Dietrich, my embodied editor.

- To Kristen Rawson for introducing me to The Neutrality Exercise.

- To all my meditation teachers: Baba Muktananda and Guru Mayi.

- To my mom Kathryn Julia, who set me on a path to self discovery from my conception.

- To everyone and anyone doing any of the work necessary for us humans to find more depth and peace while we share space on this planet together.

An Introduction to The Neutrality Exercise

The Neutrality Exercise is a playful practice that increases our emotional and psychological awareness, and challenges our responses to any topic towards which we choose to apply it. How? By tapping into our imagination to help us look at scenarios from more than one perspective.

It can be challenging to remain neutral on a topic in real time, especially when you feel perspective is based on solid research and others have opinions that are less informed. Using our imagination to walk us through various scenarios allows us time and space to process our thoughts and feelings without the pressure of real-time responses. The more we do this, the more ability we have to navigate what could otherwise be reactive situations. We increase our ability to engage in fruitful conversations and establish boundaries that allow everyone to move forward.

It is our experience that doing this exercise repeatedly:
- Decreases our tendency to react.
- Increases our ability to respond.
- Bolsters our ability to establish boundaries.

This workbook is designed to guide you into The Neutrality Exercise as a practice. Our hope is that by doing what is set forth in this workbook, you will establish your own practice. The eventual goal is to apply The Neutrality Exercise to anything you want to challenge your emotional and psychological reactions to. We share this tool with the hope that you apply it toward your own liberation.

***Because The Neutrality Exercise is designed to play with our emotional and psychological responses, be aware that you may be triggered as a result of using it. With that awareness, please be gentle with yourself before, during, and after your practice. Create sufficient space and time to complete the exercise, and be attentive to your feelings. Have your self-care already in place.

The more you practice this exercise, the more you will come to find how easily The Neutrality Exercise lends itself to the healing process of using *triggers as medicine*.

Holistic Peer Counseling (HPC)

The Neutrality Exercise is one of several exercises taught as part of a larger Holistic Peer Counseling (HPC) curriculum. Holistic Peer Counseling is Do It Yourself (DIY) technology that teaches the potentially radical perspective that distress patterns need loving attention to heal—and so we practice holding space for our peers' distress patterns. We learn how to be both a client and a counselor so that we can heal ourselves and facilitate healing for others.

Through coming to understand both sides of the counselor/client relationship, we learn tools and distinctions that help us use our personal triggers to catalyze healing—we come to use *triggers as medicine*. The peer counseling dynamic not only keeps the person being counseled in control of their session, it breaks us out of the "I am healer" and "you heal me" mindset. It acknowledges that we all have the ability to give and receive loving attention, and provides opportunities for healing as a result.

Of course, some of us are far better at giving than receiving (and vice versa), and we have myriad programmed responses to receiving attention,. For this as well as many other reasons, the peer counseling process isn't necessarily an easy one to learn; nor is it a quick-fix solution. HPC represents a chance to engage in a challenging, ongoing, life-altering practice that offers literally unimaginable rewards to those who are ready for change.

If you are interested in learning more about HPC, registration is always open at www.holisticpeercounseling.com.

Our textbook is also available on amazon: **Holistic Peer Counseling**.

Getting Started with The Neutrality Exercise

In the beginning, it will serve you to be very intentional about practicing The Neutrality Exercise. As you build up some facility with the tool, you will find you may start practicing in the context of living your life, in real time, almost without noticing.

Because this series is designed for the beginner, we will provide very specific directions. Of course, you can take or leave any directions we may offer.

1—Create the space and time you need to engage in a mindful practice. Sometimes setting at timer can be useful so that you can fully engage in the practice without worrying about using up more time that you have available to you.

2—Practice these exercises in order: (They are laid out in detail on the following pages)
- A Basic Grounding
- The Neutrality Exercise
- Presencing

3—Take some time to use the Introspection pages to integrate what you learned by running through the exercise.

Prior to working The Neutrality Exercise, it is a good idea to get grounded. As such, we are including this Grounding Exercise as a method to calm your body and deepen your awareness. We suggest that you ground prior to each round of The Neutrality Exercise.

Let's begin....

Bringing Attention to Your Breath

You can sit, stand, lie down, or do whatever works best for you. Our aim is to have your body in a state of balance, release, and maybe even in a state of pleasure. If you are seated, your weight should be evenly distributed on your sit bones. If you are standing, keep your weight evenly distributed between your feet. If you are pregnant and lying down, do so on your left side with pillows to support you. If you are not pregnant and want to lie down, do so on your back, perhaps with your knees up and feet on the ground if that is more comfortable for you. Aim for comfort. Aim for relaxation. Aim for pleasure.

Once you are settled, close your eyes or bring them to a soft gaze—whichever brings relaxation to your eyes.

Now, bring your attention to your breathing. Be a witness to it. Notice. Is it fast? Is it slow? Is it deep? Is it shallow? Witness your breathing body like you would calmly witness a new baby discovering its feet for the first time. Just be with it. Feel your inhales and exhales.

You can now become a bit more active with your breath. If you feel a desire to change your breathing at all—perhaps change its rhythm—please do. Maybe you notice you would like to take a deep breath in and let out a sigh. Maybe you feel like doing a little rapid breathing to free it up. Or maybe it's all good just how it is. Just take a moment to experiment with your breath.

Once you have made any desired changes, bring yourself back to the passive witness state again. Be with your breathing. Be with your body. Be with yourself.

Grounding the Body

Bring your attention deep into your lower abdomen, focusing just in front of the spine at the core of your body. Imagine there is a cylindrical tube that attaches this point in your body to the surface of the Earth. You can imagine this tube to be whatever you choose: a hose, a root, a tree trunk, a lava tube, a ray of light. Really see it in your mind's eye and imagine it connecting the center of you with the Earth.

On your next exhale, imagine your tube sinking deeper into the Earth. It falls easily. It gets longer and longer. It falls through all the layers of the Earth. It falls through rock, water, and magma—all the way down to the very center of the Earth. Feel it as the core of your body firmly attaches to the core of Mother Earth. Your bottom is heavy and you feel your connection.

On your next exhale, imagine taking all the energy you don't need right now and sending it down through the tube. Give it to Mother Earth. You don't have to see it or know what it is, just suggest to yourself that you're letting go of whatever isn't needed right now. It is falling toward the center of the Earth. Where there is tension or pain in your body, relax the area and let it all drain into Mother Earth. This is her compost; she will take it and turn it into fertile soil.

Try to match your breathing with your release: on your inhale, gather all your undesirable energy into a blob of goo and then on your exhale, let it drop down your tube into the Earth. Or you can be more physical about it. On your inhale, stand up and tense your muscles, bringing in and intensifying the energy, and then on your exhale, release all your muscles and fall over or into your seat.

Take some time to practice this on your own for a bit, unguided. During this time, give whatever you want over to Mother Earth through your grounding cord.

Now, take a moment to stop your download and simply feel yourself, feel your grounding cord. Be with what is for a few moments. Bring your attention back to the room slowly. If your eyes are closed, open them slowly. Wiggle your body around a bit. Do what you need to do to bring your awareness back into the room and be present with the people who are here.

In this book we repeatedly offer you two versions of The Neutrality Exercise. One version is designed to take you through different scenarios while looking at a topic. The other is designed to take you through contrasting scenarios related to a topic. Below, you will find general outlines for both versions of The Neutrality Exercise.

As your practice builds, feel free to play with these outlines and create different scenarios for yourself. We give you some space to do that at the end of the book. You really can change any element of the practice to focus on anything in any way you feel will help you better investigate your emotional and psychological responses.

1. The Neutrality Exercise (Single topic: Bubbles)

Imagine you are in the presence of your stated topic. Simply be present with it. Notice how you feel and the thoughts running through my mind being present with it. Be there, be with how you are feeling, and be with the thoughts that come to your mind. (Allow 30-60secs to pass.)

Next, imagine there is a sheet of glass between you and your topic. Notice. Do your feelings change at all while you look at it through a piece of glass? Do your thoughts change? Notice how you feel and the thoughts that come to your mind while looking at your topic through a sheet of glass. (Allow 30-60secs to pass.)

Now, image you are in a huge room—think of a ballroom or a large conference room. Imagine your topic is at the opposite end of the room from you; you can see it, but from far away. Investigate how this feels and what thoughts arise. Did your reaction change at all from the prior scenarios? (Allow 30-60secs to pass.)

Now, imagine you are at the top of a tall tower and the topic is outside the tower, down on the ground. You can barely see it, but you know it is there. See what this feels like and what thoughts come to your mind. (Allow 30-60secs to pass.)

Finally, return to simply being with your topic. Be with your topic and be with how you feel and the thoughts that come to your mind. (Allow 30-60secs to pass.)

2. The Neutrality Exercise (Contrasting topics: Bubbles and no bubbles)

Imagine you are in the presence of your stated topic. Simply be present with it. with it. Notice how you feel and the thoughts running through my mind being present with your topic. Be there, be with how you are feeling, and be with the thoughts that come to your mind. (Allow 30-60secs to pass.)

Next, imagine there is a sheet of glass between you and your topic. Notice. Do your feelings or thoughts change at all while you look at your topic through a piece of glass? Notice how you feel and the thoughts that come to your mind looking at your topic through a sheet of glass. (Allow 30-60secs to pass.)

Now, image you are in a huge room—think of a ballroom or a large conference room. Imagine your topic is at the opposite end of the room from you; you can see it, but from far away. Investigate how this feels and whether your feelings or thoughts change from the prior scenarios. (Allow 30-60secs to pass.)

Now, go back to simply being with your topic. Again, simply be in its presence. Notice how you feel and what thoughts arise being there with it. Be there and be with how you are. (Allow 30-60secs to pass.)

Next, imagine you are in the presence of a contrast to your stated topic. Simply be present with the contrast to your original topic.

Notice how you feel and the thoughts that come to your mind being present with it. Be there and be with how you are. (Allow 30-60secs to pass.)

And then imagine there is a sheet of glass between you and the contrast to your topic. Notice. Do your feelings or thoughts change when you look at it through a piece of glass? Notice how you feel and the thoughts that come to your mind looking at the contrast to your topic through a sheet of glass. (Allow 30-60secs to pass.)

Now, imagine you are in a huge room. Imagine you are at the opposite end of this room from your contrasting topic; you can see it, but from far away. Investigate how this is for you and whether your thoughts or feelings change from the prior scenarios. (Allow 30-60secs to pass.)

Finally, go back to simply being with your topic. Again, simply be in its presence. Maybe notice if your imagination comes to rest more on the original topic or the contrast to it. Notice how you feel and the thoughts that come to your mind being there with whatever you find. Be there and be with how you are. (Allow 30-60secs to pass.)

Finally, go back to just being with your topic. Again, just be in its presence. Maybe notice if your imagination comes to rest more on the original topic or the contrast to it. Notice how you feel and the thoughts that come to your mind being there with whatever you find. Be there and be with how you are. (Allow 30-60secs to pass.)

Presencing

One of the most useful tools from Holistic Peer Counseling is Presencing.

When we are triggered, our attention is no longer in the present moment. Presencing brings our attention back to the present moment so that we can interact with what is happening in the here and now. We find Presencing to be a necessary tool for navigating the trigger-laden world in which we live.

A common Presencing exercise is The Senses Exercise, where we use our senses to bring ourself back to the present moment. We can pay attention to what our eyes are seeing in the space around us. We can use our ears to hear the sounds around us. We can feel the sensations on our skin or in our bodies or pay attention to the smells around us and the tastes in our mouth. Any of these actions can be powerful tools to bring us back to the present moment.

Other methods of Presencing include math problems, jokes, describing something familiar, hopping on one foot, or saying our names over and over. In truth, there are infinite methods of Presencing. If you are new to this practice, start with some of what has been suggested above. Practice often and you will come to better understand the magic of Presencing. Once you acquire some mastery, you will find methods that work best for you.

Before fully stepping away from your practice, take some moments to ponder what you learned from running through The Neutrality Exercise on your specific topic.

You can use these questions below and/or simply express yourself freely in words, patterns, art, etc.

Introspection

- How was that for you?

- What did you learn about yourself?

- Did any of your reactions surprise you?

- How will you incorporate the experience of working The Neutrality Exercise on this topic into your life?

The Entire Practice: Step by Step

1. A Basic Grounding

Bringing Attention to Your Breath

You can sit, stand, lie down, or do whatever works best for you. Our aim is to have your body in a state of balance, release, and maybe even in a state of pleasure. If you are seated, your weight should be evenly distributed on your sit bones. If you are standing, keep your weight evenly distributed between your feet. If you are pregnant and lying down, do so on your left side with pillows to support you. If you are not pregnant and want to lie down, do so on your back, perhaps with your knees up and feet on the ground if that is more comfortable for you. Aim for comfort. Aim for relaxation. Aim for pleasure.

Once you are settled, close your eyes or bring them to a soft gaze—whichever brings relaxation to your eyes.

Now, bring your attention to your breathing. Be a witness to it. Notice. Is it fast? Is it slow? Is it deep? Is it shallow? Witness your breathing body like you would calmly witness a new baby discovering its feet for the first time. Just be with it. Feel your inhales and exhales.

You can now become a bit more active with your breath. If you feel a desire to change your breathing at all—perhaps change its rhythm—please do. Maybe you notice you would like to take a deep breath in and let out a sigh. Maybe you feel like doing a little rapid breathing to free it up. Or maybe it's all good just how it is. Just take a moment to experiment with your breath.

Once you have made any desired changes, bring yourself back to the passive witness state again. Be with your breathing. Be with your body. Be with yourself.

Grounding the Body

Bring your attention deep into your lower abdomen, focusing just in front of the spine at the core of your body. Imagine there is a cylindrical tube that attaches this point in your body to the surface of the Earth. You can imagine this tube to be whatever you choose: a hose, a root, a tree trunk, a lava tube, a ray of light. Really see it in your mind's eye and imagine it connecting the center of you with the Earth.

On your next exhale, imagine your tube sinking deeper into the Earth. It falls easily. It gets longer and longer. It falls through all the layers of the Earth. It falls through rock, water, and magma—all the way down to the very center of the Earth. Feel it as the core of your body firmly attaches to the core of Mother Earth. Your bottom is heavy and you feel your connection.

On your next exhale, imagine taking all the energy you don't need right now and sending it down through the tube. Give it to Mother Earth. You don't have to see it or know what it is, just suggest to yourself that you're letting go of whatever isn't needed right now. It is falling toward the center of the Earth. Where there is tension or pain in your body, relax the area and let it all drain into Mother Earth. This is her compost; she will take it and turn it into fertile soil.

Try to match your breathing with your release: on your inhale, gather all your undesirable energy into a blob of goo and then on your exhale, let it drop down your tube into the Earth. Or you can be more physical about it. On your inhale, stand up and tense your muscles, bringing in and intensifying the energy, and then on your

exhale, release all your muscles and fall over or into your seat.

Take some time to practice this on your own for a bit, unguided. During this time, give whatever you want over to Mother Earth through your grounding cord.

Now, take a moment to stop your download and simply feel yourself, feel your grounding cord. Be with what is for a few moments. Bring your attention back to the room slowly. If your eyes are closed, open them slowly. Wiggle your body around a bit. Do what you need to do to bring your awareness back into the room and be present with the people who are here.

2. The Neutrality Exercise (A or B)

A. Example 1 (Non-contrasting)

Imagine you are in the presence of your stated topic. Simply be present with it. Notice how you feel and the thoughts running through my mind being present with it. Be there, be with how you are feeling, and be with the thoughts that come to your mind. (Allow 30-60secs to pass.)

Next, imagine there is a sheet of glass between you and your topic. Notice. Do your feelings change at all while you look at it through a piece of glass? Do your thoughts change? Notice how you feel and the thoughts that come to your mind while looking at your topic through a sheet of glass. (Allow 30-60secs to pass.)

Now, image you are in a huge room—think of a ballroom or a large conference room. Imagine your topic is at the opposite end of the room from you; you can see it, but from far away. Investigate how this feels and what thoughts arise. Did your reaction change at all from the prior scenarios? (Allow 30-60secs to pass.)

Now, imagine you are at the top of a tall tower and the topic is outside the tower, down on the ground. You can barely see it, but you know it is there. See what this feels like and what thoughts come to your mind. (Allow 30-60secs to pass.)

Finally, return to simply being with your topic. Be with your topic and be with how you feel and the thoughts that come to your mind. (Allow 30-60secs to pass.)

B. Example 2 (Contrasting)

Imagine you are in the presence of your stated topic. Simply be present with it. with it. Notice how you feel and the thoughts running through my mind being present with your topic. Be there, be with how you are feeling, and be with the thoughts that come to your mind. (Allow 30-60secs to pass.)

Next, imagine there is a sheet of glass between you and your topic. Notice. Do your feelings or thoughts change at all while you look at your topic through a piece of glass? Notice how you feel and the thoughts that come to your mind looking at your topic through a sheet of glass. (Allow 30-60secs to pass.)

Now, image you are in a huge room—think of a ballroom or a large conference room. Imagine your topic is at the opposite end of the room from you; you can see it, but from far away. Investigate how this feels and whether your feelings or thoughts change from the prior scenarios. (Allow 30-60secs to pass.)

Now, go back to simply being with your topic. Again, simply be in its presence. Notice how you feel and what thoughts arise being there with it. Be there and be with how you are. (Allow 30-60secs to pass.)

Next, imagine you are in the presence of a contrast to your stated topic. Simply be present with the contrast to your original topic. Notice how you feel and the thoughts that come to your mind being present with it. Be there and be with how you are. (Allow 30-60secs to pass.)

And then imagine there is a sheet of glass between you and the contrast to your topic. Notice. Do your feelings or thoughts change when you look at it through a piece of glass? Notice how you feel and the thoughts that come to your mind looking at the contrast to your topic through a sheet of glass. (Allow 30-60secs to pass.)

Now, imagine you are in a huge room. Imagine you are at the opposite end of this room from your contrasting topic; you can see it, but from far away. Investigate how this is for you and whether your thoughts or feelings change from the prior scenarios. (Allow 30-60secs to pass.)

Finally, go back to simply being with your topic. Again, simply be in its presence. Maybe notice if your imagination comes to rest more on the original topic or the contrast to it. Notice how you feel and the thoughts that come to your mind being there with whatever you find. Be there and be with how you are. (Allow 30-60secs to pass.)

3. Presencing

Take a moment to bring your awareness back into the present moment. Open your eyes and look around you. See what is in the space with you. Hear the sounds that are around you. Feel the air around you and the body you are living in. You can even pay attention to what you are tasting and smelling. Take some moments to bring your attention to the present moment and away from the topic you just explored.

4. Introspection

Use the following page(s) to write on what you learned about yourself by practicing The Neutrality Exercise. In particular, pay attention to anything you may have learned about your emotional attachments and biases as they relate to the topic.

Questions:

- How was that for you?

- What did you learn about yourself?

- Did any of your reactions surprise you?

- How will you incorporate the experience of working The Neutrality Exercise on this topic into your life?

Topic 1: Bubbles

We want your first round with The Neutrality Exercise to both be unrelated to the general topic of this book and be something that doesn't tend to be very triggering for people. As such, we have chosen: bubbles.

Get yourself settled and let's run through it.

1. A Basic Grounding

Bringing Attention to Your Breath

You can sit, stand, lie down, or do whatever works best for you. Our aim is to have your body in a state of balance, release, and maybe even in a state of pleasure. If you are seated, your weight should be evenly distributed on your sit bones. If you are standing, keep your weight evenly distributed between your feet. If you are pregnant and lying down, do so on your left side with pillows to support you. If you are not pregnant and want to lie down, do so on your back, perhaps with your knees up and feet on the ground if that is more comfortable for you. Aim for comfort. Aim for relaxation. Aim for pleasure.

Once you are settled, close your eyes or bring them to a soft gaze—whichever brings relaxation to your eyes.

Now, bring your attention to your breathing. Be a witness to it. Notice. Is it fast? Is it slow? Is it deep? Is it shallow? Witness your breathing body like you would calmly witness a new baby discovering its feet for the first time. Just be with it. Feel your inhales and exhales.

You can now become a bit more active with your breath. If you feel a desire to change your breathing at all—perhaps change its rhythm—please do. Maybe you notice you would like to take a deep breath in and let out a sigh. Maybe you feel like doing a little rapid breathing to free it up. Or maybe it's all good just how it is. Just take a moment to experiment with your breath.

Once you have made any desired changes, bring yourself back to the passive witness state again. Be with your breathing. Be with your body. Be with yourself.

Grounding the Body

Bring your attention deep into your lower abdomen, focusing just in front of the spine at the core of your body. Imagine there is a cylindrical tube that attaches this point in your body to the surface of the Earth. You can imagine this tube to be whatever you choose: a hose, a root, a tree trunk, a lava tube, a ray of light. Really see it in your mind's eye and imagine it connecting the center of you with the Earth.

On your next exhale, imagine your tube sinking deeper into the Earth. It falls easily. It gets longer and longer. It falls through all the layers of the Earth. It falls through rock, water, and magma—all the way down to the very center of the Earth. Feel it as the core of your body firmly attaches to the core of Mother Earth. Your bottom is heavy and you feel your connection.

On your next exhale, imagine taking all the energy you don't need right now and sending it down through the tube. Give it to Mother Earth. You don't have to see it or know what it is, just suggest to yourself that you're letting go of whatever isn't needed right now. It is falling toward the center of the Earth. Where there is tension or pain in your body, relax the area and let it all drain into Mother Earth. This is her compost; she will take it and turn it into fertile soil.

Try to match your breathing with your release: on your inhale, gather all your undesirable energy into a blob of goo and then on your exhale, let it drop down your tube into the Earth. Or you can be more physical about it. On your inhale, stand up and tense your muscles, bringing in and intensifying the energy, and then on your exhale, release all your muscles and fall over or into your seat.

Take some time to practice this on your own for a bit, unguided. During this time, give whatever you want over to Mother Earth through your grounding cord.

Now, take a moment to stop your download and simply feel yourself, feel your grounding cord. Be with what is for a few moments. Bring your attention back to the room slowly. If your eyes are closed, open them slowly. Wiggle your body around a bit. Do what you need to do to bring your awareness back into the room and be present with the people who are here.

2. The Neutrality Exercise: Bubbles

Imagine you are in the presence of bubbles. Just be there with them. Notice how it is for you to be there with bubbles. Be there with them; be with how you are feeling and the thoughts that come to your mind. (Allow 30–60 seconds to pass.)

Next, imagine there is a sheet of glass between you and bubbles. Notice. Do your feelings change at all while you look at bubbles through a sheet of glass? Do your thoughts change? Notice how you feel and the thoughts that come to your mind being with bubbles while having a sheet of glass between you and them. (Allow 30–60 seconds to pass.)

Now, imagine you are in a huge room—think of a ballroom or large conference room. Imagine the bubbles are at the opposite end of the room from you; you can see them, but from far away. Investigate how this feels and whether your feelings or thoughts change from the prior scenario. (Allow 30–60 seconds to pass.)

And now, imagine you are at the top of a tall tower and the bubbles are outside the tower, down on the ground. What does it feel like and what thoughts come to your mind when you look at bubbles far down below you? (Allow 30–60 seconds to pass.)

Finally, return to simply being with bubbles. Be with the bubbles and be with how you feel and the thoughts that come to your mind being there with them. (Allow 30–60 seconds to pass.)

3. Presence Yourself

Before you step away completely, take a moment to bring your awareness back into the present moment. Open your eyes and look around you. See what is in the space with you. Hear the sounds that are around you. Feel the air around you and the body you are living in. You can even pay attention to what you are tasting and smelling. Take some moments to bring your attention to the present moment and away from the topic you just explored.

4. Introspection

How was that for you?

What did you learn about yourself?

Did any of your reactions surprise you?

How will you bring the experience of working The Neutrality Exercise on this topic into your life?

Neutrality Exercise Workbook AAMI

Topic 2: Skin to Skin

1. A Basic Grounding

Bringing Attention to Your Breath

You can sit, stand, lie down, or do whatever works best for you. Our aim is to have your body in a state of balance, release, and maybe even in a state of pleasure. If you are seated, your weight should be evenly distributed on your sit bones. If you are standing, keep your weight evenly distributed between your feet. If you are pregnant and lying down, do so on your left side with pillows to support you. If you are not pregnant and want to lie down, do so on your back, perhaps with your knees up and feet on the ground if that is more comfortable for you. Aim for comfort. Aim for relaxation. Aim for pleasure.

Once you are settled, close your eyes or bring them to a soft gaze—whichever brings relaxation to your eyes.

Now, bring your attention to your breathing. Be a witness to it. Notice. Is it fast? Is it slow? Is it deep? Is it shallow? Witness your breathing body like you would calmly witness a new baby discovering its feet for the first time. Just be with it. Feel your inhales and exhales.

You can now become a bit more active with your breath. If you feel a desire to change your breathing at all—perhaps change its rhythm—please do. Maybe you notice you would like to take a deep breath in and let out a sigh. Maybe you feel like doing a little rapid breathing to free it up. Or maybe it's all good just how it is. Just take a moment to experiment with your breath.

Once you have made any desired changes, bring yourself back to the passive witness state again. Be with your breathing. Be with your body. Be with yourself.

Grounding the Body

Bring your attention deep into your lower abdomen, focusing just in front of the spine at the core of your body. Imagine there is a cylindrical tube that attaches this point in your body to the surface of the Earth. You can imagine this tube to be whatever you choose: a hose, a root, a tree trunk, a lava tube, a ray of light. Really see it in your mind's eye and imagine it connecting the center of you with the Earth.

On your next exhale, imagine your tube sinking deeper into the Earth. It falls easily. It gets longer and longer. It falls through all the layers of the Earth. It falls through rock, water, and magma—all the way down to the very center of the Earth. Feel it as the core of your body firmly attaches to the core of Mother Earth. Your bottom is heavy and you feel your connection.

On your next exhale, imagine taking all the energy you don't need right now and sending it down through the tube. Give it to Mother Earth. You don't have to see it or know what it is, just suggest to yourself that you're letting go of whatever isn't needed right now. It is falling toward the center of the Earth. Where there is tension or pain in your body, relax the area and let it all drain into Mother Earth. This is her compost; she will take it and turn it into fertile soil.

Try to match your breathing with your release: on your inhale, gather all your undesirable energy into a blob of goo and then on your exhale, let it drop down your tube into the Earth. Or you can be more physical about it. On your inhale, stand up and tense your muscles, bringing in and intensifying the energy, and then on your

exhale, release all your muscles and fall over or into your seat.

Take some time to practice this on your own for a bit, unguided. During this time, give whatever you want over to Mother Earth through your grounding cord.

Now, take a moment to stop your download and simply feel yourself, feel your grounding cord. Be with what is for a few moments. Bring your attention back to the room slowly. If your eyes are closed, open them slowly. Wiggle your body around a bit. Do what you need to do to bring your awareness back into the room and be present with the people who are here.

2. The Neutrality Exercise: Skin to Skin

Imagine you are in the presence of a parent and a newborn baby. Be in their presence. Notice how you feel and the thoughts that come to your mind being there with them. Be there. Be with your thoughts and be with your feelings. (Allow 30-60 seconds to pass.)

Now, notice that this parent is bare chested and their newborn has nothing on their skin whatsoever. Baby is resting nude on their parent's bare chest—skin to skin. Be in their presence. Notice how you feel and the thoughts that come to your mind being there with them. Be there. Be with your thoughts. And be with your feelings. (Allow 30-60 seconds to pass.)

Next, imagine there is a sheet of glass between you and the parent and their newborn as they lay skin to skin. Notice. Do your feelings or thoughts change when you look at them through a sheet of glass? Notice how you feel and the thoughts that come to your mind being in a room with them while having a sheet of glass between you. (Allow 30-60 seconds to pass.)

Now, imagine you are in a huge room. Imagine the newborn and their parent are resting skin to skin at the opposite end of the room from you; you can see them, but they are far away. Investigate how this is for you and whether your thoughts or feelings change from the prior scenario. (Allow 30–60 seconds to pass.)

Go back to just being in the room with the parent and their newborn. Simply be in their presence. Notice how you feel and the thoughts that come to your mind being there with them. Be there. Be with your thoughts and feelings. (Allow 30–60 seconds to pass.)

Then you come to notice that the parent and newborn are snuggling fully clothed. Be in their presence. Notice how you feel and the thoughts that come to your mind being there with them snuggling with all their clothes on. Be there. Be with your thoughts. And be with your feelings. (Allow 30–60 seconds to pass.)

Next, imagine there is a sheet of glass between you and the parent and their newborn snuggling with their clothes on. Notice. Do your feelings or thoughts change when you look at them through a sheet of glass? Notice how you feel and the thoughts that come to your mind being in the room with them while having a sheet of glass between you and them. (Allow 30–60 seconds to pass.)

Now, imagine you are in a huge room. Imagine the baby and their parent are snuggling fully clothed at the opposite end of the room from you; you can see them, but from far away. Investigate how this feels. Investigate the thoughts that enter your mind. Have either changed from the prior scenarios? (Allow 30–60 seconds to pass.)

Finally, return to simply being in the room with this parent and their newborn snuggling. Be there in the room with them. Notice how you are feeling, notice your thoughts and notice whether imagine them clothed or not clothed. Be there, and be with your thoughts and feelings. (Allow 30–60 seconds to pass.)

3. Presence Yourself

Before you step away completely, take a moment to bring your awareness back into the present moment. Open your eyes and look around you. See what is in the space with you. Hear the sounds that are around you. Feel the air around you and the body you are living in. You can even pay attention to what you are tasting and smelling. Take some moments to bring your attention to the present moment and away from the topic you just explored.

4. Introspection

How was that for you?

What did you learn about yourself?

Did any of your reactions surprise you?

How will you bring the experience of working The Neutrality Exercise on this topic into your life?

Neutrality Exercise Workbook AAMI

Topic 3: Breastfeeding

1. A Basic Grounding

Bringing Attention to Your Breath

You can sit, stand, lie down, or do whatever works best for you. Our aim is to have your body in a state of balance, release, and maybe even in a state of pleasure. If you are seated, your weight should be evenly distributed on your sit bones. If you are standing, keep your weight evenly distributed between your feet. If you are pregnant and lying down, do so on your left side with pillows to support you. If you are not pregnant and want to lie down, do so on your back, perhaps with your knees up and feet on the ground if that is more comfortable for you. Aim for comfort. Aim for relaxation. Aim for pleasure.

Once you are settled, close your eyes or bring them to a soft gaze—whichever brings relaxation to your eyes.

Now, bring your attention to your breathing. Be a witness to it. Notice. Is it fast? Is it slow? Is it deep? Is it shallow? Witness your breathing body like you would calmly witness a new baby discovering its feet for the first time. Just be with it. Feel your inhales and exhales.

You can now become a bit more active with your breath. If you feel a desire to change your breathing at all—perhaps change its rhythm—please do. Maybe you notice you would like to take a deep breath in and let out a sigh. Maybe you feel like doing a little rapid breathing to free it up. Or maybe it's all good just how it is. Just take a moment to experiment with your breath.

Once you have made any desired changes, bring yourself back to the passive witness state again. Be with your breathing. Be with your body. Be with yourself.

Grounding the Body

Bring your attention deep into your lower abdomen, focusing just in front of the spine at the core of your body. Imagine there is a cylindrical tube that attaches this point in your body to the surface of the Earth. You can imagine this tube to be whatever you choose: a hose, a root, a tree trunk, a lava tube, a ray of light. Really see it in your mind's eye and imagine it connecting the center of you with the Earth.

On your next exhale, imagine your tube sinking deeper into the Earth. It falls easily. It gets longer and longer. It falls through all the layers of the Earth. It falls through rock, water, and magma—all the way down to the very center of the Earth. Feel it as the core of your body firmly attaches to the core of Mother Earth. Your bottom is heavy and you feel your connection.

On your next exhale, imagine taking all the energy you don't need right now and sending it down through the tube. Give it to Mother Earth. You don't have to see it or know what it is, just suggest to yourself that you're letting go of whatever isn't needed right now. It is falling toward the center of the Earth. Where there is tension or pain in your body, relax the area and let it all drain into Mother Earth. This is her compost; she will take it and turn it into fertile soil.

Try to match your breathing with your release: on your inhale, gather all your undesirable energy into a blob of goo and then on your exhale, let it drop down your tube into the Earth. Or you can be more physical about it. On your inhale, stand up and tense your muscles, bringing in and intensifying the energy, and then on your

exhale, release all your muscles and fall over or into your seat.

Take some time to practice this on your own for a bit, unguided. During this time, give whatever you want over to Mother Earth through your grounding cord.

Now, take a moment to stop your download and simply feel yourself, feel your grounding cord. Be with what is for a few moments. Bring your attention back to the room slowly. If your eyes are closed, open them slowly. Wiggle your body around a bit. Do what you need to do to bring your awareness back into the room and be present with the people who are here.

2. The Neutrality Exercise: Breastfeeding

Imagine you are in the presence of a baby while it is breastfeeding. Be there with the breastfeeding team. Notice how you feel and the thoughts that come to your mind being there with them. Be with them. Be with your thoughts and be with your feelings. (Allow 30–60 seconds to pass.)

Next, imagine there is a sheet of glass between you and the breastfeeding team. Do your feelings or thoughts change? Notice how you feel and the thoughts that come to your mind watching a baby breastfeed through a sheet of glass. (Allow 30–60 seconds to pass.)

Now, imagine you are in a huge room. You sit at one end of the room. On the opposite end of the room, you know there is a baby breastfeeding. You know they are there, but you can't see them very clearly. Notice how you feel being there. Notice the thoughts that come to your mind. Be in the room with them and be with your thoughts and feelings. (Allow 30–60 seconds to pass.)

And now, imagine you are at the top of a tall tower and down on the ground below you is a baby breastfeeding. You can barely see them, but you know they are there. You are at the top of the tower and they are down below. See what it feels like and the thoughts that come to your mind imaging this scenario. (Allow 30–60 seconds to pass.)

Finally, go back to just being in the room with the breastfeeding team. Be there. Notice your thought. Notice your feelings. (Allow 30–60 seconds to pass.)

3. Presence Yourself

Before you step away completely, take a moment to bring your awareness back into the present moment. Open your eyes and look around you. See what is in the space with you. Hear the sounds that are around you. Feel the air around you and the body you are living in. You can even pay attention to what you are tasting and smelling. Take some moments to bring your attention to the present moment and away from the topic you just explored.

4. Introspection

How was that for you?

What did you learn about yourself?

Did any of your reactions surprise you?

How will you bring the experience of working The Neutrality Exercise on this topic into your life?

Neutrality Exercise Workbook AAMI

Topic 4: Hatted Newborn

1. A Basic Grounding

Bringing Attention to Your Breath

You can sit, stand, lie down, or do whatever works best for you. Our aim is to have your body in a state of balance, release, and maybe even in a state of pleasure. If you are seated, your weight should be evenly distributed on your sit bones. If you are standing, keep your weight evenly distributed between your feet. If you are pregnant and lying down, do so on your left side with pillows to support you. If you are not pregnant and want to lie down, do so on your back, perhaps with your knees up and feet on the ground if that is more comfortable for you. Aim for comfort. Aim for relaxation. Aim for pleasure.

Once you are settled, close your eyes or bring them to a soft gaze—whichever brings relaxation to your eyes.

Now, bring your attention to your breathing. Be a witness to it. Notice. Is it fast? Is it slow? Is it deep? Is it shallow? Witness your breathing body like you would calmly witness a new baby discovering its feet for the first time. Just be with it. Feel your inhales and exhales.

You can now become a bit more active with your breath. If you feel a desire to change your breathing at all—perhaps change its rhythm—please do. Maybe you notice you would like to take a deep breath in and let out a sigh. Maybe you feel like doing a little rapid breathing to free it up. Or maybe it's all good just how it is. Just take a moment to experiment with your breath.

Once you have made any desired changes, bring yourself back to the passive witness state again. Be with your breathing. Be with your body. Be with yourself.

Grounding the Body

Bring your attention deep into your lower abdomen, focusing just in front of the spine at the core of your body. Imagine there is a cylindrical tube that attaches this point in your body to the surface of the Earth. You can imagine this tube to be whatever you choose: a hose, a root, a tree trunk, a lava tube, a ray of light. Really see it in your mind's eye and imagine it connecting the center of you with the Earth.

On your next exhale, imagine your tube sinking deeper into the Earth. It falls easily. It gets longer and longer. It falls through all the layers of the Earth. It falls through rock, water, and magma—all the way down to the very center of the Earth. Feel it as the core of your body firmly attaches to the core of Mother Earth. Your bottom is heavy and you feel your connection.

On your next exhale, imagine taking all the energy you don't need right now and sending it down through the tube. Give it to Mother Earth. You don't have to see it or know what it is, just suggest to yourself that you're letting go of whatever isn't needed right now. It is falling toward the center of the Earth. Where there is tension or pain in your body, relax the area and let it all drain into Mother Earth. This is her compost; she will take it and turn it into fertile soil.

Try to match your breathing with your release: on your inhale, gather all your undesirable energy into a blob of goo and then on your exhale, let it drop down your tube into the Earth. Or you can be more physical about it. On your inhale, stand up and tense your muscles, bringing in and intensifying the energy, and then on your

exhale, release all your muscles and fall over or into your seat.

Take some time to practice this on your own for a bit, unguided. During this time, give whatever you want over to Mother Earth through your grounding cord.

Now, take a moment to stop your download and simply feel yourself, feel your grounding cord. Be with what is for a few moments. Bring your attention back to the room slowly. If your eyes are closed, open them slowly. Wiggle your body around a bit. Do what you need to do to bring your awareness back into the room and be present with the people who are here.

2. The Neutrality Exercise: Hatted Newborn

Imagine you are in the presence of a newborn baby. Be in their presence. Notice how you feel and the thoughts that come to your mind being there with them. Be there, and be with your thoughts and feelings. (Allow 30–60 seconds to pass.)

Next, notice that this newborn is wearing a hat. Be with how it is for you to be in the presence of a hatted newborn. Be there, and be with your thoughts and feelings. (Allow 30–60 seconds to pass.)

Now, imagine there is a sheet of glass between you and the hatted newborn. Do your feelings or thoughts change when you look at a hatted newborn through a sheet of glass? Notice how you feel and the thoughts that come to your mind looking at a hatted newborn through a sheet of glass. (Allow 30–60 seconds to pass.)

And now, imagine you are in a huge room. You are at one end of the room and the hatted newborn is at the opposite end of the room. You know the baby is there, but you can't see them very clearly. How is this for you? Notice if your feelings or thoughts change at all. Be with your feelings and thoughts imagining a scenario where you are at the opposite end of a large room from a hatted newborn. (Allow 30–60 seconds to pass.)

Go back to just being in the room with a newborn baby. Again, just be in their presence. Notice how you feel and the thoughts that come to your mind being there with them. Be there, and be with your thoughts and feelings. (Allow 30–60 seconds to pass.)

This time you notice that the newborn is not wearing a hat. Be in their presence. How is it for you to be in the presence of an unhatted newborn? Do your feelings or thoughts change when you imagine this scenario? Be there with the unhatted newborn. Be with your thoughts and be with your feelings. (Allow 30–60 seconds to pass.)

Next, imagine there is a sheet of glass between you and the unhatted newborn. Notice. Do your feelings or thoughts change when you look at them through a sheet of glass? Notice how you feel and the thoughts that come to your mind looking at an unhatted newborn through a sheet of glass. (Allow 30–60 seconds to pass.)

Now, imagine you are in a huge room with an unhatted newborn. You can see the newborn, but from quite far away. Investigate how it is for you and whether your thoughts or feelings change from the prior scenario. (Allow 30–60 seconds to pass.)

Finally, return to simply being with a newborn. Be there with them; notice how you are feeling and the thoughts that come to your mind. Also, notice whether you imagine the newborn with or without a hat. Be there, and be with your thoughts and feelings. (Allow 30–60 seconds to pass.)

3. Presence Yourself

Before you step away completely, take a moment to bring your awareness back into the present moment. Open your eyes and look around you. See what is in the space with you. Hear the sounds that are around you. Feel the air around you and the body you are living in. You can even pay attention to what you are tasting and smelling. Take some moments to bring your attention to the present moment and away from the topic you just explored.

4. Introspection

How was that for you?

What did you learn about yourself?

Did any of your reactions surprise you?

How will you bring the experience of working The Neutrality Exercise on this topic into your life?

Neutrality Exercise Workbook AAMI

Topic 5: Gender Scan

1. A Basic Grounding

Bringing Attention to Your Breath

You can sit, stand, lie down, or do whatever works best for you. Our aim is to have your body in a state of balance, release, and maybe even in a state of pleasure. If you are seated, your weight should be evenly distributed on your sit bones. If you are standing, keep your weight evenly distributed between your feet. If you are pregnant and lying down, do so on your left side with pillows to support you. If you are not pregnant and want to lie down, do so on your back, perhaps with your knees up and feet on the ground if that is more comfortable for you. Aim for comfort. Aim for relaxation. Aim for pleasure.

Once you are settled, close your eyes or bring them to a soft gaze—whichever brings relaxation to your eyes.

Now, bring your attention to your breathing. Be a witness to it. Notice. Is it fast? Is it slow? Is it deep? Is it shallow? Witness your breathing body like you would calmly witness a new baby discovering its feet for the first time. Just be with it. Feel your inhales and exhales.

You can now become a bit more active with your breath. If you feel a desire to change your breathing at all—perhaps change its rhythm—please do. Maybe you notice you would like to take a deep breath in and let out a sigh. Maybe you feel like doing a little rapid breathing to free it up. Or maybe it's all good just how it is. Just take a moment to experiment with your breath.

Once you have made any desired changes, bring yourself back to the passive witness state again. Be with your breathing. Be with your body. Be with yourself.

Grounding the Body

Bring your attention deep into your lower abdomen, focusing just in front of the spine at the core of your body. Imagine there is a cylindrical tube that attaches this point in your body to the surface of the Earth. You can imagine this tube to be whatever you choose: a hose, a root, a tree trunk, a lava tube, a ray of light. Really see it in your mind's eye and imagine it connecting the center of you with the Earth.

On your next exhale, imagine your tube sinking deeper into the Earth. It falls easily. It gets longer and longer. It falls through all the layers of the Earth. It falls through rock, water, and magma—all the way down to the very center of the Earth. Feel it as the core of your body firmly attaches to the core of Mother Earth. Your bottom is heavy and you feel your connection.

On your next exhale, imagine taking all the energy you don't need right now and sending it down through the tube. Give it to Mother Earth. You don't have to see it or know what it is, just suggest to yourself that you're letting go of whatever isn't needed right now. It is falling toward the center of the Earth. Where there is tension or pain in your body, relax the area and let it all drain into Mother Earth. This is her compost; she will take it and turn it into fertile soil.

Try to match your breathing with your release: on your inhale, gather all your undesirable energy into a blob of goo and then on your exhale, let it drop down your tube into the Earth. Or you can be more physical about it. On your inhale, stand up and tense your muscles, bringing in and intensifying the energy, and then on your

exhale, release all your muscles and fall over or into your seat.

Take some time to practice this on your own for a bit, unguided. During this time, give whatever you want over to Mother Earth through your grounding cord.

Now, take a moment to stop your download and simply feel yourself, feel your grounding cord. Be with what is for a few moments. Bring your attention back to the room slowly. If your eyes are closed, open them slowly. Wiggle your body around a bit. Do what you need to do to bring your awareness back into the room and be present with the people who are here.

2. The Neutrality Exercise: Gender Scan

Imagine you are in the presence of someone who is pregnant. Be in their presence. Notice how you feel and the thoughts that come to your mind being there with them. Be there, and be with your thoughts and feelings. (Allow 30–60 seconds to pass.)

Now, notice that this pregnant person is having an ultrasound to determine the baby's gender (gender scan). How is it for you to imagine being with someone pregnant undergoing a gender scan? Imagine this scenario and be present to your thoughts and feelings. (Allow 30–60 seconds to pass.)

Next, imagine there is a sheet of glass between you and someone pregnant undergoing a gender scan. Do your feelings or thoughts change when you look at them through a sheet of glass? Notice how you feel and the thoughts that come to your mind being present with a pregnant person undergoing a gender scan while having a sheet of glass between them and you. (Allow 30–60 seconds to pass.)

Now, imagine you are in a huge room. At one end of this room is a pregnant person undergoing a gender scan. You are at the opposite end of the room. You know they are there, but you can't see them very clearly. How is this for you? Notice if your feelings or thoughts change at all from the prior scenarios. Be with your thoughts and feelings imagining a scenario where you are at the opposite end of a large room from a pregnant person undergoing a gender scan. (Allow 30–60 seconds to pass.)

And now, imagine you are at the top of a tall tower and down on the ground below you is a pregnant person undergoing a gender scan. See what it feels like and the thoughts that come to your mind when you imagine a scenario where you are at the top of a tall tower looking down on a pregnant person undergoing a gender scan. (Allow 30–60 seconds to pass.)

Finally, go back to just being in the room with a pregnant person. Simply be in their presence. Notice how you feel and the thoughts that come to your mind being there with them. Be there. Be with your thoughts. And be with your feelings. (Allow 30–60 seconds to pass.)

3. Presence Yourself

Before you step away completely, take a moment to bring your awareness back into the present moment. Open your eyes and look around you. See what is in the space with you. Hear the sounds that are around you. Feel the air around you and the body you are living in. You can even pay attention to what you are tasting and smelling. Take some moments to bring your attention to the present moment and away from the topic you just explored.

4. Introspection

How was that for you?

What did you learn about yourself?

Did any of your reactions surprise you?

How will you bring the experience of working The Neutrality Exercise on this topic into your life?

Neutrality Exercise Workbook AAMI

Topic 6: Preceptors

1. A Basic Grounding

Bringing Attention to Your Breath

You can sit, stand, lie down, or do whatever works best for you. Our aim is to have your body in a state of balance, release, and maybe even in a state of pleasure. If you are seated, your weight should be evenly distributed on your sit bones. If you are standing, keep your weight evenly distributed between your feet. If you are pregnant and lying down, do so on your left side with pillows to support you. If you are not pregnant and want to lie down, do so on your back, perhaps with your knees up and feet on the ground if that is more comfortable for you. Aim for comfort. Aim for relaxation. Aim for pleasure.

Once you are settled, close your eyes or bring them to a soft gaze—whichever brings relaxation to your eyes.

Now, bring your attention to your breathing. Be a witness to it. Notice. Is it fast? Is it slow? Is it deep? Is it shallow? Witness your breathing body like you would calmly witness a new baby discovering its feet for the first time. Just be with it. Feel your inhales and exhales.

You can now become a bit more active with your breath. If you feel a desire to change your breathing at all—perhaps change its rhythm—please do. Maybe you notice you would like to take a deep breath in and let out a sigh. Maybe you feel like doing a little rapid breathing to free it up. Or maybe it's all good just how it is. Just take a moment to experiment with your breath.

Once you have made any desired changes, bring yourself back to the passive witness state again. Be with your breathing. Be with your body. Be with yourself.

Grounding the Body

Bring your attention deep into your lower abdomen, focusing just in front of the spine at the core of your body. Imagine there is a cylindrical tube that attaches this point in your body to the surface of the Earth. You can imagine this tube to be whatever you choose: a hose, a root, a tree trunk, a lava tube, a ray of light. Really see it in your mind's eye and imagine it connecting the center of you with the Earth.

On your next exhale, imagine your tube sinking deeper into the Earth. It falls easily. It gets longer and longer. It falls through all the layers of the Earth. It falls through rock, water, and magma—all the way down to the very center of the Earth. Feel it as the core of your body firmly attaches to the core of Mother Earth. Your bottom is heavy and you feel your connection.

On your next exhale, imagine taking all the energy you don't need right now and sending it down through the tube. Give it to Mother Earth. You don't have to see it or know what it is, just suggest to yourself that you're letting go of whatever isn't needed right now. It is falling toward the center of the Earth. Where there is tension or pain in your body, relax the area and let it all drain into Mother Earth. This is her compost; she will take it and turn it into fertile soil.

Try to match your breathing with your release: on your inhale, gather all your undesirable energy into a blob of goo and then on your exhale, let it drop down your tube into the Earth. Or you can be more physical about it. On your inhale, stand up and tense your muscles, bringing in and intensifying the energy, and then on your

exhale, release all your muscles and fall over or into your seat.

Take some time to practice this on your own for a bit, unguided. During this time, give whatever you want over to Mother Earth through your grounding cord.

Now, take a moment to stop your download and simply feel yourself, feel your grounding cord. Be with what is for a few moments. Bring your attention back to the room slowly. If your eyes are closed, open them slowly. Wiggle your body around a bit. Do what you need to do to bring your awareness back into the room and be present with the people who are here.

2. The Neutrality Exercise: Preceptors

Imagine you are in the presence of a preceptor. Be in their presence. Notice how you feel and the thoughts that come to your mind being there with them. Be there, and be with your thoughts and feelings. (Allow 30–60 seconds to pass.)

Now, notice that the preceptor is doing things you don't agree with. Be with how you feel and the thoughts that come to your mind imagining yourself in the presence of a preceptor doing things differently than you think they should be done. Be there, and be with your thoughts and feelings. (Allow 30–60 seconds to pass.)

Next, imagine there is a sheet of glass between you and the preceptor as they do things differently than you think they should be done. Notice. Do your feelings or thoughts change when you look at them through a sheet of glass? Notice how you feel and the thoughts that come to your mind watching a preceptor through a sheet of glass as they do things differently than you think they should be done. (Allow 30–60 seconds to pass.)

Now, imagine you are in a huge room. Imagine the preceptor is at the opposite end of the room from you doing things differently than you think they should be done. You can see them, but they are far away. Investigate how this feels. Investigate your thoughts that arise. Notice whether anything changes for you compared to when you imagined the prior scenarios. (Allow 30–60 seconds to pass.)

Go back to just being present with a preceptor again. Imagine being in their presence. Notice how you feel and the thoughts that come to your mind being there with them. Be there. Be with your thoughts. And be with your feelings. (Allow 30–60 seconds to pass.)

Now, come to notice that the preceptor is doing everything exactly the way you think they should be done. Be in their presence. Notice how you feel and the thoughts that come to your mind being there with a preceptor as they do everything exactly the way you think they should be done. Be there, and be with your thoughts and feelings. (Allow 30–60 seconds to pass.)

Next, imagine there is a sheet of glass between you and the preceptor doing everything exactly the way you think they should be done. Notice. Do your feelings change when you look at them through a sheet of glass? Notice how you feel and the thoughts that come to your mind watching a preceptor through a sheet of glass as they do everything exactly how you think they should be done. (Allow 30–60 seconds to pass.)

Now, imagine you are in a huge room. The preceptor is doing everything you think they should be doing on one end of the room and you are on the opposite end of the room. You can barely see them, but you know they are doing everything the way you think they should be done. Investigate how this feels. Investigate the thoughts that arise in your mind. Has anything changed within you since pondering the prior scenarios? (Allow 30–60 seconds to pass.)

Finally, return to simply being with a preceptor. Imagine being there with them; notice how you are feeling and the thoughts that come to your mind. Also notice which scenario your mind comes to rest upon: a preceptor who does everything just how you think they should be done or one who does nothing the way you think they should be done. Be there, and be with your thoughts and feelings. (Allow 30–60 seconds to pass.)

3. Presence Yourself

Before you step away completely, take a moment to bring your awareness back into the present moment. Open your eyes and look around you. See what is in the space with you. Hear the sounds that are around you. Feel the air around you and the body you are living in. You can even pay attention to what you are tasting and smelling. Take some moments to bring your attention to the present moment and away from the topic you just explored.

4. Introspection

How was that for you?

What did you learn about yourself?

Did any of your reactions surprise you?

How will you bring the experience of working The Neutrality Exercise on this topic into your life?

Topic 7: Baby Baths

1. A Basic Grounding

Bringing Attention to Your Breath

You can sit, stand, lie down, or do whatever works best for you. Our aim is to have your body in a state of balance, release, and maybe even in a state of pleasure. If you are seated, your weight should be evenly distributed on your sit bones. If you are standing, keep your weight evenly distributed between your feet. If you are pregnant and lying down, do so on your left side with pillows to support you. If you are not pregnant and want to lie down, do so on your back, perhaps with your knees up and feet on the ground if that is more comfortable for you. Aim for comfort. Aim for relaxation. Aim for pleasure.

Once you are settled, close your eyes or bring them to a soft gaze—whichever brings relaxation to your eyes.

Now, bring your attention to your breathing. Be a witness to it. Notice. Is it fast? Is it slow? Is it deep? Is it shallow? Witness your breathing body like you would calmly witness a new baby discovering its feet for the first time. Just be with it. Feel your inhales and exhales.

You can now become a bit more active with your breath. If you feel a desire to change your breathing at all—perhaps change its rhythm—please do. Maybe you notice you would like to take a deep breath in and let out a sigh. Maybe you feel like doing a little rapid breathing to free it up. Or maybe it's all good just how it is. Just take a moment to experiment with your breath.

Once you have made any desired changes, bring yourself back to the passive witness state again. Be with your breathing. Be with your body. Be with yourself.

Grounding the Body

Bring your attention deep into your lower abdomen, focusing just in front of the spine at the core of your body. Imagine there is a cylindrical tube that attaches this point in your body to the surface of the Earth. You can imagine this tube to be whatever you choose: a hose, a root, a tree trunk, a lava tube, a ray of light. Really see it in your mind's eye and imagine it connecting the center of you with the Earth.

On your next exhale, imagine your tube sinking deeper into the Earth. It falls easily. It gets longer and longer. It falls through all the layers of the Earth. It falls through rock, water, and magma—all the way down to the very center of the Earth. Feel it as the core of your body firmly attaches to the core of Mother Earth. Your bottom is heavy and you feel your connection.

On your next exhale, imagine taking all the energy you don't need right now and sending it down through the tube. Give it to Mother Earth. You don't have to see it or know what it is, just suggest to yourself that you're letting go of whatever isn't needed right now. It is falling toward the center of the Earth. Where there is tension or pain in your body, relax the area and let it all drain into Mother Earth. This is her compost; she will take it and turn it into fertile soil.

Try to match your breathing with your release: on your inhale, gather all your undesirable energy into a blob of goo and then on your exhale, let it drop down your tube into the Earth. Or you can be more physical about it. On your inhale, stand up and tense your muscles, bringing in and intensifying the energy, and then on your

exhale, release all your muscles and fall over or into your seat.

Take some time to practice this on your own for a bit, unguided. During this time, give whatever you want over to Mother Earth through your grounding cord.

Now, take a moment to stop your download and simply feel yourself, feel your grounding cord. Be with what is for a few moments. Bring your attention back to the room slowly. If your eyes are closed, open them slowly. Wiggle your body around a bit. Do what you need to do to bring your awareness back into the room and be present with the people who are here.

2. The Neutrality Exercise: Baby Baths

Imagine you are in the presence of a newborn baby. Be in their presence. Notice how you feel and the thoughts that come to your mind being there with them. Be there, and be with your thoughts and feelings. (Allow 30–60 seconds to pass.)

Now, notice that this newborn is being placed into a baby bath. Be with how it is for you to be in the presence of a newborn getting a baby bath. Be there. Be with your thoughts and be with your feelings. (Allow 30–60 seconds to pass.)

Next, imagine there is a sheet of glass between you and the newborn getting a baby bath. Do your feelings or thoughts change when you look at a baby bath through a sheet of glass? Notice how you feel and the thoughts that come to your mind watching a baby bath through a sheet of glass. (Allow 30–60 seconds to pass.)

Now, imagine you are in a huge room. You are at one end of this room and the newborn receiving a baby bath is at the opposite end of the room. You know they are there, but you can't see them very clearly. How is this for you? Notice if your thoughts or feelings change at all. Be with your thoughts and feelings imagining a scenario where you are at the opposite end of a large room from a newborn receiving a baby bath. (Allow 30–60 seconds to pass.)

And now, imagine you are at the top of a tall tower and down on the ground below you is a newborn receiving a baby bath. See what it feels like and notice the thoughts that come to your mind imaging a scenario where you are at the top of a tall tower, looking down on the newborn receiving a baby bath far below you. (Allow 30–60 seconds to pass.)

Finally, go back to simply being present with a newborn baby. Again, just be in their presence. Notice how you feel and the thoughts that come to your mind being there with them. Be there, and be with your thoughts and feelings. (Allow 30–60 seconds to pass.)

3. Presence Yourself

Before you step away completely, take a moment to bring your awareness back into the present moment. Open your eyes and look around you. See what is in the space with you. Hear the sounds that are around you. Feel the air around you and the body you are living in. You can even pay attention to what you are tasting and smelling. Take some moments to bring your attention to the present moment and away from the topic you just explored.

4. Introspection

How was that for you?

What did you learn about yourself?

Did any of your reactions surprise you?

How will you bring the experience of working The Neutrality Exercise on this topic into your life?

Neutrality Exercise Workbook AAMI

Topic 8: Monitoring

1. A Basic Grounding

Bringing Attention to Your Breath

You can sit, stand, lie down, or do whatever works best for you. Our aim is to have your body in a state of balance, release, and maybe even in a state of pleasure. If you are seated, your weight should be evenly distributed on your sit bones. If you are standing, keep your weight evenly distributed between your feet. If you are pregnant and lying down, do so on your left side with pillows to support you. If you are not pregnant and want to lie down, do so on your back, perhaps with your knees up and feet on the ground if that is more comfortable for you. Aim for comfort. Aim for relaxation. Aim for pleasure.

Once you are settled, close your eyes or bring them to a soft gaze—whichever brings relaxation to your eyes.

Now, bring your attention to your breathing. Be a witness to it. Notice. Is it fast? Is it slow? Is it deep? Is it shallow? Witness your breathing body like you would calmly witness a new baby discovering its feet for the first time. Just be with it. Feel your inhales and exhales.

You can now become a bit more active with your breath. If you feel a desire to change your breathing at all—perhaps change its rhythm—please do. Maybe you notice you would like to take a deep breath in and let out a sigh. Maybe you feel like doing a little rapid breathing to free it up. Or maybe it's all good just how it is. Just take a moment to experiment with your breath.

Once you have made any desired changes, bring yourself back to the passive witness state again. Be with your breathing. Be with your body. Be with yourself.

Grounding the Body

Bring your attention deep into your lower abdomen, focusing just in front of the spine at the core of your body. Imagine there is a cylindrical tube that attaches this point in your body to the surface of the Earth. You can imagine this tube to be whatever you choose: a hose, a root, a tree trunk, a lava tube, a ray of light. Really see it in your mind's eye and imagine it connecting the center of you with the Earth.

On your next exhale, imagine your tube sinking deeper into the Earth. It falls easily. It gets longer and longer. It falls through all the layers of the Earth. It falls through rock, water, and magma—all the way down to the very center of the Earth. Feel it as the core of your body firmly attaches to the core of Mother Earth. Your bottom is heavy and you feel your connection.

On your next exhale, imagine taking all the energy you don't need right now and sending it down through the tube. Give it to Mother Earth. You don't have to see it or know what it is, just suggest to yourself that you're letting go of whatever isn't needed right now. It is falling toward the center of the Earth. Where there is tension or pain in your body, relax the area and let it all drain into Mother Earth. This is her compost; she will take it and turn it into fertile soil.

Try to match your breathing with your release: on your inhale, gather all your undesirable energy into a blob of goo and then on your exhale, let it drop down your tube into the Earth. Or you can be more physical about it. On your inhale, stand up and tense your muscles, bringing in and intensifying the energy, and then on your

exhale, release all your muscles and fall over or into your seat.

Take some time to practice this on your own for a bit, unguided. During this time, give whatever you want over to Mother Earth through your grounding cord.

Now, take a moment to stop your download and simply feel yourself, feel your grounding cord. Be with what is for a few moments. Bring your attention back to the room slowly. If your eyes are closed, open them slowly. Wiggle your body around a bit. Do what you need to do to bring your awareness back into the room and be present with the people who are here.

2. The Neutrality Exercise: Monitoring

Imagine you are in the presence of someone in labor. Be in their presence. Notice how you feel and the thoughts that come to your mind being there with them. Be there. Be with your thoughts. And be with your feelings. (Allow 30–60 seconds to pass.)

Now, notice that some hours have gone by and no one has come to monitor the fetus. Be there with this person in labor knowing that no one has come to monitor the fetus in a number of hours. Imagine this scenario and be with whatever feelings or thoughts may arise. (Allow 30–60 seconds to pass.)

Next, imagine you are in a huge room. And imagine that you have been witnessing this labor for hours from across a huge room, no one has come to monitor the fetus. Be with your feelings and thoughts as you imagine this scenario. (Allow 30–60 seconds to pass.)

Go back to simply being present with someone in labor. Be there with them, be with how you are feeling, and be with any thoughts that may arise. (Allow 30–60 seconds to pass.)

This time, you notice that the person in labor is hooked up to a continuous fetal monitor. Again, be there with them, and notice your feelings and thoughts as you witness them laboring attached to a continuous fetal monitor. (Allow 30–60 seconds to pass.)

Next, imagine you are in a huge room. Imagine that you are witnessing someone in labor, connected to a continuous fetal monitor, far away on the other side of the room from you. Be with your feelings and thoughts as you imagine this scenario. (Allow 30–60 seconds to pass.)

Go back to simply being present with someone in labor. Be there with them, be with how you are feeling, and be with any thoughts that may arise. (Allow 30–60 seconds to pass.)

Now, notice that about an hour has gone by and someone has come in to monitor the fetus for some moments. Imagine this scenario where you have been with someone in labor for an hour and someone comes in to monitor the fetus for some moments. Be with this scenario in your mind and be with whatever feelings or thoughts may arise. (Allow 30–60 seconds to pass.)

Next, imagine you are in a huge room. Imagine that you have been witnessing this labor for an hour from across this huge room and someone comes in to monitor the fetus for some moments. Be with your feelings and thoughts as you imagine this scenario. (Allow 30–60 seconds to pass.)

Finally, go back to simply being present with someone in labor. Imagine being in their presence. Notice how you feel and the thoughts that come to your mind being there with them. Also, notice which scenario your mind comes to rest upon: no monitoring, continuous monitoring, or intermittent monitoring. Be there, and be with your thoughts and feelings. (Allow 30–60 seconds to pass.)

3. Presence Yourself

Before you step away completely, take a moment to bring your awareness back into the present moment. Open your eyes and look around you. See what is in the space with you. Hear the sounds that are around you. Feel the air around you and the body you are living in. You can even pay attention to what you are tasting and smelling. Take some moments to bring your attention to the present moment and away from the topic you just explored.

4. Introspection

How was that for you?

What did you learn about yourself?

Did any of your reactions surprise you?

How will you bring the experience of working The Neutrality Exercise on this topic into your life?

Neutrality Exercise Workbook AAMI

Topic 9: Formula

1. A Basic Grounding

Bringing Attention to Your Breath

You can sit, stand, lie down, or do whatever works best for you. Our aim is to have your body in a state of balance, release, and maybe even in a state of pleasure. If you are seated, your weight should be evenly distributed on your sit bones. If you are standing, keep your weight evenly distributed between your feet. If you are pregnant and lying down, do so on your left side with pillows to support you. If you are not pregnant and want to lie down, do so on your back, perhaps with your knees up and feet on the ground if that is more comfortable for you. Aim for comfort. Aim for relaxation. Aim for pleasure.

Once you are settled, close your eyes or bring them to a soft gaze—whichever brings relaxation to your eyes.

Now, bring your attention to your breathing. Be a witness to it. Notice. Is it fast? Is it slow? Is it deep? Is it shallow? Witness your breathing body like you would calmly witness a new baby discovering its feet for the first time. Just be with it. Feel your inhales and exhales.

You can now become a bit more active with your breath. If you feel a desire to change your breathing at all—perhaps change its rhythm—please do. Maybe you notice you would like to take a deep breath in and let out a sigh. Maybe you feel like doing a little rapid breathing to free it up. Or maybe it's all good just how it is. Just take a moment to experiment with your breath.

Once you have made any desired changes, bring yourself back to the passive witness state again. Be with your breathing. Be with your body. Be with yourself.

Grounding the Body

Bring your attention deep into your lower abdomen, focusing just in front of the spine at the core of your body. Imagine there is a cylindrical tube that attaches this point in your body to the surface of the Earth. You can imagine this tube to be whatever you choose: a hose, a root, a tree trunk, a lava tube, a ray of light. Really see it in your mind's eye and imagine it connecting the center of you with the Earth.

On your next exhale, imagine your tube sinking deeper into the Earth. It falls easily. It gets longer and longer. It falls through all the layers of the Earth. It falls through rock, water, and magma—all the way down to the very center of the Earth. Feel it as the core of your body firmly attaches to the core of Mother Earth. Your bottom is heavy and you feel your connection.

On your next exhale, imagine taking all the energy you don't need right now and sending it down through the tube. Give it to Mother Earth. You don't have to see it or know what it is, just suggest to yourself that you're letting go of whatever isn't needed right now. It is falling toward the center of the Earth. Where there is tension or pain in your body, relax the area and let it all drain into Mother Earth. This is her compost; she will take it and turn it into fertile soil.

Try to match your breathing with your release: on your inhale, gather all your undesirable energy into a blob of goo and then on your exhale, let it drop down your tube into the Earth. Or you can be more physical about it. On your inhale, stand up and tense your muscles, bringing in and intensifying the energy, and then on your

exhale, release all your muscles and fall over or into your seat.

Take some time to practice this on your own for a bit, unguided. During this time, give whatever you want over to Mother Earth through your grounding cord.

Now, take a moment to stop your download and simply feel yourself, feel your grounding cord. Be with what is for a few moments. Bring your attention back to the room slowly. If your eyes are closed, open them slowly. Wiggle your body around a bit. Do what you need to do to bring your awareness back into the room and be present with the people who are here.

2. The Neutrality Exercise: Formula

Imagine you are in the presence of a baby. Be in their presence. Notice how you feel being there with them. Be there, and be with your thoughts and feelings. (Allow 30–60 seconds to pass.)

Now, notice that someone begins to formula feed the baby. Be in their presence. Notice how you feel being there with them. Be there, and be with your thoughts and feelings. (Allow 30–60 seconds to pass.)

Next, imagine there is a sheet of glass between you and the baby being formula fed. Notice. Do your feelings change when you look at them through a sheet of glass? Notice what it is like for you to watch through a sheet of glass as a baby is being formula fed. Notice your thoughts and feelings. (Allow 30–60 seconds to pass.)

Now, imagine you are in a huge room. Imagine that you are at one end of the room and on the opposite end of the room there is a baby being formula fed. You can see them, but they are far away. Notice how this is for you and whether your feelings or thoughts change from the prior scenarios. (Allow 30–60 seconds to pass.)

And now, imagine you are at the top of a tall tower and down on the ground below you is a baby being formula fed. See what it feels like and what thoughts arise as you imagine a scenario where you are at the top of a tall tower looking down below at a baby being formula fed. Notice the feelings and thoughts that arise as you imagine. (Allow 30–60 seconds to pass.)

Finally, return to simply being with a baby. Be there with them. Notice your thoughts. Notice your feelings. Be with it all. (Allow 30–60 seconds to pass.)

3. Presence Yourself

Before you step away completely, take a moment to bring your awareness back into the present moment. Open your eyes and look around you. See what is in the space with you. Hear the sounds that are around you. Feel the air around you and the body you are living in. You can even pay attention to what you are tasting and smelling. Take some moments to bring your attention to the present moment and away from the topic you just explored.

4. Introspection

How was that for you?

What did you learn about yourself?

Did any of your reactions surprise you?

How will you bring the experience of working The Neutrality Exercise on this topic into your life?

Neutrality Exercise Workbook AAMI

Topic 10: Circumcision

1. A Basic Grounding

Bringing Attention to Your Breath

You can sit, stand, lie down, or do whatever works best for you. Our aim is to have your body in a state of balance, release, and maybe even in a state of pleasure. If you are seated, your weight should be evenly distributed on your sit bones. If you are standing, keep your weight evenly distributed between your feet. If you are pregnant and lying down, do so on your left side with pillows to support you. If you are not pregnant and want to lie down, do so on your back, perhaps with your knees up and feet on the ground if that is more comfortable for you. Aim for comfort. Aim for relaxation. Aim for pleasure.

Once you are settled, close your eyes or bring them to a soft gaze—whichever brings relaxation to your eyes.

Now, bring your attention to your breathing. Be a witness to it. Notice. Is it fast? Is it slow? Is it deep? Is it shallow? Witness your breathing body like you would calmly witness a new baby discovering its feet for the first time. Just be with it. Feel your inhales and exhales.

You can now become a bit more active with your breath. If you feel a desire to change your breathing at all—perhaps change its rhythm—please do. Maybe you notice you would like to take a deep breath in and let out a sigh. Maybe you feel like doing a little rapid breathing to free it up. Or maybe it's all good just how it is. Just take a moment to experiment with your breath.

Once you have made any desired changes, bring yourself back to the passive witness state again. Be with your breathing. Be with your body. Be with yourself.

Grounding the Body

Bring your attention deep into your lower abdomen, focusing just in front of the spine at the core of your body. Imagine there is a cylindrical tube that attaches this point in your body to the surface of the Earth. You can imagine this tube to be whatever you choose: a hose, a root, a tree trunk, a lava tube, a ray of light. Really see it in your mind's eye and imagine it connecting the center of you with the Earth.

On your next exhale, imagine your tube sinking deeper into the Earth. It falls easily. It gets longer and longer. It falls through all the layers of the Earth. It falls through rock, water, and magma—all the way down to the very center of the Earth. Feel it as the core of your body firmly attaches to the core of Mother Earth. Your bottom is heavy and you feel your connection.

On your next exhale, imagine taking all the energy you don't need right now and sending it down through the tube. Give it to Mother Earth. You don't have to see it or know what it is, just suggest to yourself that you're letting go of whatever isn't needed right now. It is falling toward the center of the Earth. Where there is tension or pain in your body, relax the area and let it all drain into Mother Earth. This is her compost; she will take it and turn it into fertile soil.

Try to match your breathing with your release: on your inhale, gather all your undesirable energy into a blob of goo and then on your exhale, let it drop down your tube into the Earth. Or you can be more physical about it. On your inhale, stand up and tense your muscles, bringing in and intensifying the energy, and then on your

exhale, release all your muscles and fall over or into your seat.

Take some time to practice this on your own for a bit, unguided. During this time, give whatever you want over to Mother Earth through your grounding cord.

Now, take a moment to stop your download and simply feel yourself, feel your grounding cord. Be with what is for a few moments. Bring your attention back to the room slowly. If your eyes are closed, open them slowly. Wiggle your body around a bit. Do what you need to do to bring your awareness back into the room and be present with the people who are here.

2. The Neutrality Exercise: Circumcision

Imagine you are sitting with a family awaiting the birth of their child. Be with them. Notice how you feel and the thoughts that come to your mind being there with them. Be there. Be with your thoughts and be with your feelings. (Allow 30–60 seconds to pass.)

Now, notice that the conversation moves to the topic of circumcision. They are trying to decide whether they will circumcise their child. Again, just be present to this imagined scenario. Notice how you feel and the thoughts that arise in your mind being there with them as they discuss the prospect of circumcising their child. (Allow 30–60 seconds to pass.)

Next, imagine there is a sheet of glass between you and a family discussing whether to circumcise their child. Notice. Do your feelings or thoughts change when you look at them through a sheet of glass? Notice how you feel and the thoughts that come to your mind watching through a sheet of glass as a family decides whether to circumcise their child. (Allow 30–60 seconds to pass.)

Remove the glass and be there with them discussing circumcision. They start to lean toward the decision to have their child circumcised. Notice how hearing this feels for you. What thoughts begin to enter your mind? Take some moments to be with your thoughts and feelings. (Allow 30–60 seconds to pass.)

Place the sheet of glass back between you and the family as they seem to lean toward the decision to have their child circumcised. Does having a sheet of glass between you change your thoughts or feelings? Again, take some time to be with your thoughts and feelings as you sit on the other side of a sheet of glass from a family discussing their desire to have their child circumcised. (Allow 30–60 seconds to pass.)

Now, return to simply being with this family awaiting the birth of their child. Just be with them. There is no particular discussion happening. Just be with them in your imagination and notice your thoughts and feelings. (Allow 30–60 seconds to pass.)

Again, the conversation moves to the topic of circumcision. Now they start to speak as though they will choose not to have their child circumcised. Notice how it is for you to be with a family opting not to have their child circumcised. Be with your thoughts and feelings. (Allow 30–60 seconds to pass.)

And now, place a sheet of glass between you and the family again as they seem to lean toward the decision to not have their child circumcised. Does having a sheet of glass between you and them change how you feel or the thoughts that arise in your mind? Again, take some time to be with your thoughts and feelings as you sit on the other side of a sheet of glass from a family discussing their desire to not have their child circumcised. (Allow 30–60 seconds to pass.)

Finally, return to simply being in the room with this family expecting a baby. Be there in the room with them. Notice how you are feeling and whether you find your mind bringing you to any of the above scenarios. Be there. Be with your thoughts and be with your feelings. (Allow 30–60 seconds to pass.)

3. Presence Yourself

Before you step away completely, take a moment to bring your awareness back into the present moment. Open your eyes and look around you. See what is in the space with you. Hear the sounds that are around you. Feel the air around you and the body you are living in. You can even pay attention to what you are tasting and smelling. Take some moments to bring your attention to the present moment and away from the topic you just explored.

4. Introspection

How was that for you?

What did you learn about yourself?

Did any of your reactions surprise you?

How will you bring the experience of working The Neutrality Exercise on this topic into your life?

Neutrality Exercise Workbook AAMI

Topic 11: Schedule a Caesarean

1. A Basic Grounding

Bringing Attention to Your Breath

You can sit, stand, lie down, or do whatever works best for you. Our aim is to have your body in a state of balance, release, and maybe even in a state of pleasure. If you are seated, your weight should be evenly distributed on your sit bones. If you are standing, keep your weight evenly distributed between your feet. If you are pregnant and lying down, do so on your left side with pillows to support you. If you are not pregnant and want to lie down, do so on your back, perhaps with your knees up and feet on the ground if that is more comfortable for you. Aim for comfort. Aim for relaxation. Aim for pleasure.

Once you are settled, close your eyes or bring them to a soft gaze—whichever brings relaxation to your eyes.

Now, bring your attention to your breathing. Be a witness to it. Notice. Is it fast? Is it slow? Is it deep? Is it shallow? Witness your breathing body like you would calmly witness a new baby discovering its feet for the first time. Just be with it. Feel your inhales and exhales.

You can now become a bit more active with your breath. If you feel a desire to change your breathing at all—perhaps change its rhythm—please do. Maybe you notice you would like to take a deep breath in and let out a sigh. Maybe you feel like doing a little rapid breathing to free it up. Or maybe it's all good just how it is. Just take a moment to experiment with your breath.

Once you have made any desired changes, bring yourself back to the passive witness state again. Be with your breathing. Be with your body. Be with yourself.

Grounding the Body

Bring your attention deep into your lower abdomen, focusing just in front of the spine at the core of your body. Imagine there is a cylindrical tube that attaches this point in your body to the surface of the Earth. You can imagine this tube to be whatever you choose: a hose, a root, a tree trunk, a lava tube, a ray of light. Really see it in your mind's eye and imagine it connecting the center of you with the Earth.

On your next exhale, imagine your tube sinking deeper into the Earth. It falls easily. It gets longer and longer. It falls through all the layers of the Earth. It falls through rock, water, and magma—all the way down to the very center of the Earth. Feel it as the core of your body firmly attaches to the core of Mother Earth. Your bottom is heavy and you feel your connection.

On your next exhale, imagine taking all the energy you don't need right now and sending it down through the tube. Give it to Mother Earth. You don't have to see it or know what it is, just suggest to yourself that you're letting go of whatever isn't needed right now. It is falling toward the center of the Earth. Where there is tension or pain in your body, relax the area and let it all drain into Mother Earth. This is her compost; she will take it and turn it into fertile soil.

Try to match your breathing with your release: on your inhale, gather all your undesirable energy into a blob of goo and then on your exhale, let it drop down your tube into the Earth. Or you can be more physical about it. On your inhale, stand up and tense your muscles, bringing in and intensifying the energy, and then on your

exhale, release all your muscles and fall over or into your seat.

Take some time to practice this on your own for a bit, unguided. During this time, give whatever you want over to Mother Earth through your grounding cord.

Now, take a moment to stop your download and simply feel yourself, feel your grounding cord. Be with what is for a few moments. Bring your attention back to the room slowly. If your eyes are closed, open them slowly. Wiggle your body around a bit. Do what you need to do to bring your awareness back into the room and be present with the people who are here.

2. The Neutrality Exercise: Scheduled a Caesarean

Imagine you are with a family awaiting the birth of their child. Be in their presence. Notice how you feel and the thoughts that come to your mind being there with them. Be there. Be with your thoughts. And be with your feelings. (Allow 30–60 seconds to pass.)

Notice that their provider is suggesting to them that they schedule a caesarean. Notice how this is for you. Take some moments to imagine you are with an expecting family whose provider is suggesting that they schedule a caesarean. Be with them. And be with your thoughts and feelings. (Allow 30–60 seconds to pass.)

Next, imagine there is a sheet of glass between you and the expecting family as their provider suggests that they schedule a caesarean. Notice. Do your thoughts or feelings change when you watch them through a sheet of glass? Notice how it is for you to watch through a sheet of glass as a provider suggests to a family that they schedule a caesarean. (Allow 30–60 seconds to pass.)

Now, imagine you are in a huge room. At one end of this room is an expecting family whose provider is suggesting that they schedule a caesarean. You are on the opposite end of the room. You can see them, but they are far away. Investigate how this feels and what thoughts come to your mind. Does anything change for you from the prior scenarios? (Allow 30–60 seconds to pass.)

And now, imagine you are at the top of a tall tower and down on the ground below you is an expecting family whose provider is suggesting that they schedule a caesarean. From the top of the tower, see them far below. Witness your thoughts and feelings. Are they different than during the prior scenarios? (Allow 30–60 seconds to pass.)

Finally, return to simply being with the expecting family. Be with them. Notice how you are feeling and what thoughts arise in your mind. (Allow 30–60 seconds to pass.)

3. Presence Yourself

Before you step away completely, take a moment to bring your awareness back into the present moment. Open your eyes and look around you. See what is in the space with you. Hear the sounds that are around you. Feel the air around you and the body you are living in. You can even pay attention to what you are tasting and smelling. Take some moments to bring your attention to the present moment and away from the topic you just explored.

4. Introspection

How was that for you?

What did you learn about yourself?

Did any of your reactions surprise you?

How will you bring the experience of working The Neutrality Exercise on this topic into your life?

Neutrality Exercise Workbook AAMI

Topic 12: Local Obstetricians (OB)

1. A Basic Grounding

Bringing Attention to Your Breath

You can sit, stand, lie down, or do whatever works best for you. Our aim is to have your body in a state of balance, release, and maybe even in a state of pleasure. If you are seated, your weight should be evenly distributed on your sit bones. If you are standing, keep your weight evenly distributed between your feet. If you are pregnant and lying down, do so on your left side with pillows to support you. If you are not pregnant and want to lie down, do so on your back, perhaps with your knees up and feet on the ground if that is more comfortable for you. Aim for comfort. Aim for relaxation. Aim for pleasure.

Once you are settled, close your eyes or bring them to a soft gaze—whichever brings relaxation to your eyes.

Now, bring your attention to your breathing. Be a witness to it. Notice. Is it fast? Is it slow? Is it deep? Is it shallow? Witness your breathing body like you would calmly witness a new baby discovering its feet for the first time. Just be with it. Feel your inhales and exhales.

You can now become a bit more active with your breath. If you feel a desire to change your breathing at all—perhaps change its rhythm—please do. Maybe you notice you would like to take a deep breath in and let out a sigh. Maybe you feel like doing a little rapid breathing to free it up. Or maybe it's all good just how it is. Just take a moment to experiment with your breath.

Once you have made any desired changes, bring yourself back to the passive witness state again. Be with your breathing. Be with your body. Be with yourself.

Grounding the Body

Bring your attention deep into your lower abdomen, focusing just in front of the spine at the core of your body. Imagine there is a cylindrical tube that attaches this point in your body to the surface of the Earth. You can imagine this tube to be whatever you choose: a hose, a root, a tree trunk, a lava tube, a ray of light. Really see it in your mind's eye and imagine it connecting the center of you with the Earth.

On your next exhale, imagine your tube sinking deeper into the Earth. It falls easily. It gets longer and longer. It falls through all the layers of the Earth. It falls through rock, water, and magma—all the way down to the very center of the Earth. Feel it as the core of your body firmly attaches to the core of Mother Earth. Your bottom is heavy and you feel your connection.

On your next exhale, imagine taking all the energy you don't need right now and sending it down through the tube. Give it to Mother Earth. You don't have to see it or know what it is, just suggest to yourself that you're letting go of whatever isn't needed right now. It is falling toward the center of the Earth. Where there is tension or pain in your body, relax the area and let it all drain into Mother Earth. This is her compost; she will take it and turn it into fertile soil.

Try to match your breathing with your release: on your inhale, gather all your undesirable energy into a blob of goo and then on your exhale, let it drop down your tube into the Earth. Or you can be more physical about it. On your inhale, stand up and tense your muscles, bringing in and intensifying the energy, and then on your

exhale, release all your muscles and fall over or into your seat.

Take some time to practice this on your own for a bit, unguided. During this time, give whatever you want over to Mother Earth through your grounding cord.

Now, take a moment to stop your download and simply feel yourself, feel your grounding cord. Be with what is for a few moments. Bring your attention back to the room slowly. If your eyes are closed, open them slowly. Wiggle your body around a bit. Do what you need to do to bring your awareness back into the room and be present with the people who are here.

2. The Neutrality Exercise: Local Obstetricians (OB)

Imagine you are in the presence of a local obstetrician (OB). Be in their presence. Notice how you feel and what thoughts arise in your mind being there with them. Be there. Be with your thoughts. And be with your feelings. (Allow 30–60 seconds to pass.)

Next, imagine there is a sheet of glass between you and the local OB. Notice. Do your feelings or thoughts change when you look at them through a sheet of glass? Notice how you feel and the thoughts that come to your mind being with the local OB when there is a sheet of glass between the two of you. (Allow 30–60 seconds to pass.)

Now, imagine you are in a huge room. Imagine the local OB is at the opposite end of the room from you. You can see them, but they are far away. Investigate how this feels. Investigate your thoughts. And notice whether your thoughts or feelings change from the prior scenarios. (Allow 30–60 seconds to pass.)

And now, imagine you are at the top of a tall tower and the local OB is down on the ground below you. You are at the top of the tower. See the local OB far below you. Do your thoughts change? Do your feelings change? Be with your thoughts and feelings as you ponder this scenario. (Allow 30–60 seconds to pass.)

Finally, return to simply being in the room with the local OB. Be there in the room with them and notice how it is for you. Be there. Be with your thoughts and be with your feelings. (Allow 30–60 seconds to pass.)

3. Presence Yourself

Before you step away completely, take a moment to bring your awareness back into the present moment. Open your eyes and look around you. See what is in the space with you. Hear the sounds that are around you. Feel the air around you and the body you are living in. You can even pay attention to what you are tasting and smelling. Take some moments to bring your attention to the present moment and away from the topic you just explored.

4. Introspection

How was that for you?

What did you learn about yourself?

Did any of your reactions surprise you?

How will you bring the experience of working The Neutrality Exercise on this topic into your life?

Neutrality Exercise Workbook AAMI

Topic 13: You Choose

1. A Basic Grounding

Bringing Attention to Your Breath

You can sit, stand, lie down, or do whatever works best for you. Our aim is to have your body in a state of balance, release, and maybe even in a state of pleasure. If you are seated, your weight should be evenly distributed on your sit bones. If you are standing, keep your weight evenly distributed between your feet. If you are pregnant and lying down, do so on your left side with pillows to support you. If you are not pregnant and want to lie down, do so on your back, perhaps with your knees up and feet on the ground if that is more comfortable for you. Aim for comfort. Aim for relaxation. Aim for pleasure.

Once you are settled, close your eyes or bring them to a soft gaze—whichever brings relaxation to your eyes.

Now, bring your attention to your breathing. Be a witness to it. Notice. Is it fast? Is it slow? Is it deep? Is it shallow? Witness your breathing body like you would calmly witness a new baby discovering its feet for the first time. Just be with it. Feel your inhales and exhales.

You can now become a bit more active with your breath. If you feel a desire to change your breathing at all—perhaps change its rhythm—please do. Maybe you notice you would like to take a deep breath in and let out a sigh. Maybe you feel like doing a little rapid breathing to free it up. Or maybe it's all good just how it is. Just take a moment to experiment with your breath.

Once you have made any desired changes, bring yourself back to the passive witness state again. Be with your breathing. Be with your body. Be with yourself.

Grounding the Body

Bring your attention deep into your lower abdomen, focusing just in front of the spine at the core of your body. Imagine there is a cylindrical tube that attaches this point in your body to the surface of the Earth. You can imagine this tube to be whatever you choose: a hose, a root, a tree trunk, a lava tube, a ray of light. Really see it in your mind's eye and imagine it connecting the center of you with the Earth.

On your next exhale, imagine your tube sinking deeper into the Earth. It falls easily. It gets longer and longer. It falls through all the layers of the Earth. It falls through rock, water, and magma—all the way down to the very center of the Earth. Feel it as the core of your body firmly attaches to the core of Mother Earth. Your bottom is heavy and you feel your connection.

On your next exhale, imagine taking all the energy you don't need right now and sending it down through the tube. Give it to Mother Earth. You don't have to see it or know what it is, just suggest to yourself that you're letting go of whatever isn't needed right now. It is falling toward the center of the Earth. Where there is tension or pain in your body, relax the area and let it all drain into Mother Earth. This is her compost; she will take it and turn it into fertile soil.

Try to match your breathing with your release: on your inhale, gather all your undesirable energy into a blob of goo and then on your exhale, let it drop down your tube into the Earth. Or you can be more physical about it. On your inhale, stand up and tense your muscles, bringing in and intensifying the energy, and then on your

exhale, release all your muscles and fall over or into your seat.

Take some time to practice this on your own for a bit, unguided. During this time, give whatever you want over to Mother Earth through your grounding cord.

Now, take a moment to stop your download and simply feel yourself, feel your grounding cord. Be with what is for a few moments. Bring your attention back to the room slowly. If your eyes are closed, open them slowly. Wiggle your body around a bit. Do what you need to do to bring your awareness back into the room and be present with the people who are here.

2. The Neutrality Exercise - Pick a topic and write it here:

Use one of the scripts below or write your own.

A. The Neutrality Exercise:

Imagine you are in the presence of your stated topic. Just be in a room with it. Notice how you feel being in a room with it. Be there and be with how you are feeling and the thoughts that come to your mind. (Allow 30-60secs to pass.)

Next, imagine there is a sheet of glass between you and your topic. Notice. Do your feelings change at all while you look at it through a sheet of glass? DO your thoughts change? Notice how you feel and the thoughts that come to your mind being in the room with it while having a sheet of glass between you and it. (Allow 30-60secs to pass.)

Now, image you are in a huge room - think of a ball room or large conference room. Imagine your topic is at the opposite end of the

room from you; you can see it, but from far away. Investigate how this feels and what thoughts arise. Did your reaction change at all from the prior scenarios. (Allow 30-60secs to pass.)

Now imagine you are at the top of a tall tower and the topic is outside the tower, down on the ground. You can barely see it but you know it is there. See what this feels like and what thoughts come to your mind. (Allow 30-60secs to pass.)

Finally, return to simply being with your topic. Be with your topic and be with how you feel and the thoughts that come to your mind. (Allow 30-60secs to pass.)

B. The Neutrality Exercise (Contrasting):

Imagine you are in the presence of your stated topic. Just be in a room with it. Notice how you feel being in a room with it. Be there and be with how you are feeling and the thoughts that come to your mind. (Allow 30-60secs to pass.)

Next, imagine there is a sheet of glass between you and your topic. Notice. Do your feelings change at all while you look at it through a sheet of glass? Notice how you feel and the thoughts that come to your mind being in the room with it while having a sheet of glass between you and it. (Allow 30-60secs to pass.)

Now, image you are in a huge room - think of a ball room or large conference room. Imagine your topic is at the opposite end of the room from you; you can see it, but from far away. Investigate how this feels and whether your feelings or thoughts change from the prior scenarios. (Allow 30-60secs to pass.)

Now, go back to just being your topic. Again, just be in its presence. Notice how you feel and what thoughts arise being there with it. Be

there and be with how you are. (Allow 30-60secs to pass.)

Next, imagine you are in the presence of a contrast to your stated topic. Just be in a room with it. Notice how you feel and the thoughts that come to your mind being in a room with it. Be there and be with how you are. (Allow 30-60secs to pass.)

And then imagine there is a sheet of glass between you and the contrast to your topic. Notice. Do your feelings or thoughts change when you look at it through a sheet of glass? Notice how you feel and the thoughts that come to your mind being in the room with it while having a sheet of glass between you and it. (Allow 30-60secs to pass.)

Now, image you are in a huge room. Imagine you are at the opposite end of this large room from your contrasting topic; you can see it, but from far away. Investigate how this is for you and whether your thoughts or feelings change from the prior scenarios. (Allow 30-60secs to pass.)

Finally, go back to just being your topic. Again, just be in its presence. Maybe notice if your imagination comes to rest more on the original topic or the contrast to it. Notice how you feel and the thoughts that come to your mind being there with whichever you find. Be there and be with how you are. (Allow 30-60secs to pass.)

3. Presence Yourself

Before you step away completely, take a moment to bring your awareness back into the present moment. Open your eyes and look around you. See what is in the space with you. Hear the sounds that are around you. Feel the air around you and the body you are living in. You can even pay attention to what you are tasting and smelling.

Neutrality Exercise Workbook AAMI

Take some moments to bring your attention to the present moment and away from the topic you just explored.

4. Introspection

How was that for you?

What did you learn about yourself?

Did any of your reactions surprise you?

How will you bring the experience of working The Neutrality Exercise on this topic into your life?

Neutrality Exercise Workbook AAMI

Topic 14: You Choose

1. A Basic Grounding

Bringing Attention to Your Breath

You can sit, stand, lie down, or do whatever works best for you. Our aim is to have your body in a state of balance, release, and maybe even in a state of pleasure. If you are seated, your weight should be evenly distributed on your sit bones. If you are standing, keep your weight evenly distributed between your feet. If you are pregnant and lying down, do so on your left side with pillows to support you. If you are not pregnant and want to lie down, do so on your back, perhaps with your knees up and feet on the ground if that is more comfortable for you. Aim for comfort. Aim for relaxation. Aim for pleasure.

Once you are settled, close your eyes or bring them to a soft gaze—whichever brings relaxation to your eyes.

Now, bring your attention to your breathing. Be a witness to it. Notice. Is it fast? Is it slow? Is it deep? Is it shallow? Witness your breathing body like you would calmly witness a new baby discovering its feet for the first time. Just be with it. Feel your inhales and exhales.

You can now become a bit more active with your breath. If you feel a desire to change your breathing at all—perhaps change its rhythm—please do. Maybe you notice you would like to take a deep breath in and let out a sigh. Maybe you feel like doing a little rapid breathing to free it up. Or maybe it's all good just how it is. Just take a moment to experiment with your breath.

Once you have made any desired changes, bring yourself back to the passive witness state again. Be with your breathing. Be with your body. Be with yourself.

Grounding the Body

Bring your attention deep into your lower abdomen, focusing just in front of the spine at the core of your body. Imagine there is a cylindrical tube that attaches this point in your body to the surface of the Earth. You can imagine this tube to be whatever you choose: a hose, a root, a tree trunk, a lava tube, a ray of light. Really see it in your mind's eye and imagine it connecting the center of you with the Earth.

On your next exhale, imagine your tube sinking deeper into the Earth. It falls easily. It gets longer and longer. It falls through all the layers of the Earth. It falls through rock, water, and magma—all the way down to the very center of the Earth. Feel it as the core of your body firmly attaches to the core of Mother Earth. Your bottom is heavy and you feel your connection.

On your next exhale, imagine taking all the energy you don't need right now and sending it down through the tube. Give it to Mother Earth. You don't have to see it or know what it is, just suggest to yourself that you're letting go of whatever isn't needed right now. It is falling toward the center of the Earth. Where there is tension or pain in your body, relax the area and let it all drain into Mother Earth. This is her compost; she will take it and turn it into fertile soil.

Try to match your breathing with your release: on your inhale, gather all your undesirable energy into a blob of goo and then on your exhale, let it drop down your tube into the Earth. Or you can be more physical about it. On your inhale, stand up and tense your muscles, bringing in and intensifying the energy, and then on your

exhale, release all your muscles and fall over or into your seat.

Take some time to practice this on your own for a bit, unguided. During this time, give whatever you want over to Mother Earth through your grounding cord.

Now, take a moment to stop your download and simply feel yourself, feel your grounding cord. Be with what is for a few moments. Bring your attention back to the room slowly. If your eyes are closed, open them slowly. Wiggle your body around a bit. Do what you need to do to bring your awareness back into the room and be present with the people who are here.

2. The Neutrality Exercise - Pick a topic and write it here:

Use one of the scripts below or write your own.

A. The Neutrality Exercise:

Imagine you are in the presence of your stated topic. Just be in a room with it. Notice how you feel being in a room with it. Be there and be with how you are feeling and the thoughts that come to your mind. (Allow 30-60secs to pass.)

Next, imagine there is a sheet of glass between you and your topic. Notice. Do your feelings change at all while you look at it through a sheet of glass? DO your thoughts change? Notice how you feel and the thoughts that come to your mind being in the room with it while having a sheet of glass between you and it. (Allow 30-60secs to pass.)

Now, image you are in a huge room - think of a ball room or large conference room. Imagine your topic is at the opposite end of the

room from you; you can see it, but from far away. Investigate how this feels and what thoughts arise. Did your reaction change at all from the prior scenarios. (Allow 30-60secs to pass.)

Now imagine you are at the top of a tall tower and the topic is outside the tower, down on the ground. You can barely see it but you know it is there. See what this feels like and what thoughts come to your mind. (Allow 30-60secs to pass.)

Finally, return to simply being with your topic. Be with your topic and be with how you feel and the thoughts that come to your mind. (Allow 30-60secs to pass.)

B. The Neutrality Exercise (Contrasting):

Imagine you are in the presence of your stated topic. Just be in a room with it. Notice how you feel being in a room with it. Be there and be with how you are feeling and the thoughts that come to your mind. (Allow 30-60secs to pass.)

Next, imagine there is a sheet of glass between you and your topic. Notice. Do your feelings change at all while you look at it through a sheet of glass? Notice how you feel and the thoughts that come to your mind being in the room with it while having a sheet of glass between you and it. (Allow 30-60secs to pass.)

Now, image you are in a huge room - think of a ball room or large conference room. Imagine your topic is at the opposite end of the room from you; you can see it, but from far away. Investigate how this feels and whether your feelings or thoughts change from the prior scenarios. (Allow 30-60secs to pass.)

Now, go back to just being your topic. Again, just be in its presence. Notice how you feel and what thoughts arise being there with it. Be

there and be with how you are. (Allow 30-60secs to pass.)

Next, imagine you are in the presence of a contrast to your stated topic. Just be in a room with it. Notice how you feel and the thoughts that come to your mind being in a room with it. Be there and be with how you are. (Allow 30-60secs to pass.)

And then imagine there is a sheet of glass between you and the contrast to your topic. Notice. Do your feelings or thoughts change when you look at it through a sheet of glass? Notice how you feel and the thoughts that come to your mind being in the room with it while having a sheet of glass between you and it. (Allow 30-60secs to pass.)

Now, image you are in a huge room. Imagine you are at the opposite end of this large room from your contrasting topic; you can see it, but from far away. Investigate how this is for you and whether your thoughts or feelings change from the prior scenarios. (Allow 30-60secs to pass.)

Finally, go back to just being your topic. Again, just be in its presence. Maybe notice if your imagination comes to rest more on the original topic or the contrast to it. Notice how you feel and the thoughts that come to your mind being there with whichever you find. Be there and be with how you are. (Allow 30-60secs to pass.)

3. Presence Yourself

Before you step away completely, take a moment to bring your awareness back into the present moment. Open your eyes and look around you. See what is in the space with you. Hear the sounds that are around you. Feel the air around you and the body you are living in. You can even pay attention to what you are tasting and smelling.

Take some moments to bring your attention to the present moment and away from the topic you just explored.

4. Introspection

How was that for you?

What did you learn about yourself?

Did any of your reactions surprise you?

How will you bring the experience of working The Neutrality Exercise on this topic into your life?

Neutrality Exercise Workbook AAMI

Topic 15: You Choose

1. A Basic Grounding

Bringing Attention to Your Breath

You can sit, stand, lie down, or do whatever works best for you. Our aim is to have your body in a state of balance, release, and maybe even in a state of pleasure. If you are seated, your weight should be evenly distributed on your sit bones. If you are standing, keep your weight evenly distributed between your feet. If you are pregnant and lying down, do so on your left side with pillows to support you. If you are not pregnant and want to lie down, do so on your back, perhaps with your knees up and feet on the ground if that is more comfortable for you. Aim for comfort. Aim for relaxation. Aim for pleasure.

Once you are settled, close your eyes or bring them to a soft gaze—whichever brings relaxation to your eyes.

Now, bring your attention to your breathing. Be a witness to it. Notice. Is it fast? Is it slow? Is it deep? Is it shallow? Witness your breathing body like you would calmly witness a new baby discovering its feet for the first time. Just be with it. Feel your inhales and exhales.

You can now become a bit more active with your breath. If you feel a desire to change your breathing at all—perhaps change its rhythm—please do. Maybe you notice you would like to take a deep breath in and let out a sigh. Maybe you feel like doing a little rapid breathing to free it up. Or maybe it's all good just how it is. Just take a moment to experiment with your breath.

Once you have made any desired changes, bring yourself back to the passive witness state again. Be with your breathing. Be with your body. Be with yourself.

Grounding the Body

Bring your attention deep into your lower abdomen, focusing just in front of the spine at the core of your body. Imagine there is a cylindrical tube that attaches this point in your body to the surface of the Earth. You can imagine this tube to be whatever you choose: a hose, a root, a tree trunk, a lava tube, a ray of light. Really see it in your mind's eye and imagine it connecting the center of you with the Earth.

On your next exhale, imagine your tube sinking deeper into the Earth. It falls easily. It gets longer and longer. It falls through all the layers of the Earth. It falls through rock, water, and magma—all the way down to the very center of the Earth. Feel it as the core of your body firmly attaches to the core of Mother Earth. Your bottom is heavy and you feel your connection.

On your next exhale, imagine taking all the energy you don't need right now and sending it down through the tube. Give it to Mother Earth. You don't have to see it or know what it is, just suggest to yourself that you're letting go of whatever isn't needed right now. It is falling toward the center of the Earth. Where there is tension or pain in your body, relax the area and let it all drain into Mother Earth. This is her compost; she will take it and turn it into fertile soil.

Try to match your breathing with your release: on your inhale, gather all your undesirable energy into a blob of goo and then on your exhale, let it drop down your tube into the Earth. Or you can be more physical about it. On your inhale, stand up and tense your muscles, bringing in and intensifying the energy, and then on your

exhale, release all your muscles and fall over or into your seat.

Take some time to practice this on your own for a bit, unguided. During this time, give whatever you want over to Mother Earth through your grounding cord.

Now, take a moment to stop your download and simply feel yourself, feel your grounding cord. Be with what is for a few moments. Bring your attention back to the room slowly. If your eyes are closed, open them slowly. Wiggle your body around a bit. Do what you need to do to bring your awareness back into the room and be present with the people who are here.

2. The Neutrality Exercise - Pick a topic and write it here:

Use one of the scripts below or write your own.

A. The Neutrality Exercise:

Imagine you are in the presence of your stated topic. Just be in a room with it. Notice how you feel being in a room with it. Be there and be with how you are feeling and the thoughts that come to your mind. (Allow 30-60secs to pass.)

Next, imagine there is a sheet of glass between you and your topic. Notice. Do your feelings change at all while you look at it through a sheet of glass? DO your thoughts change? Notice how you feel and the thoughts that come to your mind being in the room with it while having a sheet of glass between you and it. (Allow 30-60secs to pass.)

Now, image you are in a huge room - think of a ball room or large conference room. Imagine your topic is at the opposite end of the

room from you; you can see it, but from far away. Investigate how this feels and what thoughts arise. Did your reaction change at all from the prior scenarios. (Allow 30-60secs to pass.)

Now imagine you are at the top of a tall tower and the topic is outside the tower, down on the ground. You can barely see it but you know it is there. See what this feels like and what thoughts come to your mind. (Allow 30-60secs to pass.)

Finally, return to simply being with your topic. Be with your topic and be with how you feel and the thoughts that come to your mind. (Allow 30-60secs to pass.)

B. The Neutrality Exercise (Contrasting):

Imagine you are in the presence of your stated topic. Just be in a room with it. Notice how you feel being in a room with it. Be there and be with how you are feeling and the thoughts that come to your mind. (Allow 30-60secs to pass.)

Next, imagine there is a sheet of glass between you and your topic. Notice. Do your feelings change at all while you look at it through a sheet of glass? Notice how you feel and the thoughts that come to your mind being in the room with it while having a sheet of glass between you and it. (Allow 30-60secs to pass.)

Now, image you are in a huge room - think of a ball room or large conference room. Imagine your topic is at the opposite end of the room from you; you can see it, but from far away. Investigate how this feels and whether your feelings or thoughts change from the prior scenarios. (Allow 30-60secs to pass.)

Now, go back to just being your topic. Again, just be in its presence. Notice how you feel and what thoughts arise being there with it. Be

there and be with how you are. (Allow 30-60secs to pass.)

Next, imagine you are in the presence of a contrast to your stated topic. Just be in a room with it. Notice how you feel and the thoughts that come to your mind being in a room with it. Be there and be with how you are. (Allow 30-60secs to pass.)

And then imagine there is a sheet of glass between you and the contrast to your topic. Notice. Do your feelings or thoughts change when you look at it through a sheet of glass? Notice how you feel and the thoughts that come to your mind being in the room with it while having a sheet of glass between you and it. (Allow 30-60secs to pass.)

Now, image you are in a huge room. Imagine you are at the opposite end of this large room from your contrasting topic; you can see it, but from far away. Investigate how this is for you and whether your thoughts or feelings change from the prior scenarios. (Allow 30-60secs to pass.)

Finally, go back to just being your topic. Again, just be in its presence. Maybe notice if your imagination comes to rest more on the original topic or the contrast to it. Notice how you feel and the thoughts that come to your mind being there with whichever you find. Be there and be with how you are. (Allow 30-60secs to pass.)

3. Presence Yourself

Before you step away completely, take a moment to bring your awareness back into the present moment. Open your eyes and look around you. See what is in the space with you. Hear the sounds that are around you. Feel the air around you and the body you are living in. You can even pay attention to what you are tasting and smelling.

Take some moments to bring your attention to the present moment and away from the topic you just explored.

Neutrality Exercise Workbook AAMI

4. Introspection

How was that for you?

What did you learn about yourself?

Did any of your reactions surprise you?

How will you bring the experience of working The Neutrality Exercise on this topic into your life?

Neutrality Exercise Workbook AAMI

Bonus Practice: Analyzing Bias

Now that you have completed this workbook, take some moments to ponder bias as it relates to The Neutrality Exercise.

Do you feel like doing The Neutrality Exercise has helped you to see your own biases better?

How is it for you to think about your biases?

Do you believe The Neutrality Exercise will change anything about how you show up in the world?

Thank you!

We too have done this work. For that reason, we know how challenging it can be.

We also know the potential we can harness together when we all do this kind of work.

So thank you from us to you for being willing to use your time and attention to become just that much more aware of who you are.

If you are interested in doing more, visit
www.holisticpeercounseling.com.

A Note From The Author

I am not the creator of The Neutrality Exercise. In truth, I am unsure of who is. It was first brought to my attention by Kristen Rawson in their version of Holistic Peer Counseling which they called Holistic Peer Support. Likewise, the concept of grounding to the center of the earth is not my brain child. This idea has roots in many traditions and was first brought into my awareness by Teri Ciacchi.

All of that said, it is through the countless hours of Siddha Yoga devotional practice I partook in as a child that I learned the power of meditative practice. I bring that experience to this book and these practices.

Likewise, it is my mother, Kathryn Julia who made the point of raising me in the world of embodiment. It is through embodiment that she continues to find healing and recovery from the violent abuse of her childhood. Learning to live IN her body has brought her recovery. As such, she raised me to use my own body as a medium for empowerment and healing. I bring these tools to this book.

Finally, a big thank you to my husband, my children and those who work with me. Each of you continues to help me and my work evolve. I love you all <3.